# To Nurse Means to Nurture
## Part Two
### The Parent Role of the Nurse with All Ages of Patients

Brian Gene Evans

## Preface

The "nurse patient relationship" as I have seen in my research is in fact a "mother and child" relationship where the nurse is supposed to act as a mother to their patient and comfort and console them in their fear and pain and that includes touching them and letting them touch you. Many patients are afraid of their nurses being impersonal when they go into a hospital setting. Yet, the ill adult patient is supposed to be allowed to regress and be able to act like a child in childlike ways and be able to make childlike requests to their nurses and be treated like a child and have their childlike needs met. And, if at some point a patient should offend a nurse by saying or doing something they don't like or just take the wrong way the nurse is supposed to figure out why the patient is saying or doing what they are saying or doing based on their own individuality before they make assumptions. In my case, I am not asking your forgiveness for asking to meet my list of needs, what I am asking forgiveness for is saying things or asking things that may offend you that are associated with other hang-ups I have that are not included on my list of needs. My list of needs have to be met. I have to have the chipper acting female nurses and the hugs and the head rubs and hand holds through needle sticks. I'm not referring to this. I am referring to being willing to forgive me for any hang-ups I bother you with that are not on my list of needs. Sometimes nurses have ideal patients and other times they have what they consider difficult patients that may offend them or even annoy them. A nurse's acceptance of the patient as a person requires that the nurse demonstrate a genuine appreciation of the patient's situation rather than looking at this behavior by itself and reacting to it without attempting to understand what prompts the behavior. When this does happen the nurse is supposed to blow it over and try to figure out a way they can handle a patient and adjust to their frame of thinking. They are to forgive them and act in the same friendly way toward them the way they always have showing them the same comfort and compassion toward them that they showed them before they even got upset with them. They are still to care for and about those patients they consider to be difficult. This book is about forgiveness, advocacy, and personalized care in the inpatient hospital setting by the nurse.

Genuine feelings of caring and acceptance are important in a helpful relationship, accompanied by a sincere desire to attempt to understand why the patient is acting as he is and then be helpful. People with autism can sometimes display odd behaviors or say or do odd things to you that may not be what they seem. Before you judge find out what causes these behaviors and what sensory issues this person may have that causes these behaviors.

Some of the odd things they say, do, or even ask of you may not be what they look like and may be misinterpreted for mischievous forms of behavior when in fact what they are thinking or feeling is something of an innocent nature that is hard for anyone to explain or understand because it is different from what you may consider to be the norm for that behavior. There are some things I nearly mentioned in this book I was so worried how you would take that I left them out just in case there was a nurse that flat wouldn't understand me about them. I figured some nurses would understand the things I nearly mentioned I left out of this book, but I also figured there would be others that would about flip if they knew what I wanted to say to them regarding some of the hang-ups I have they may not already know about yet. The things I wanted to mention are childish in nature due to my Autism but when one bases the same things on what a normal person would say, ask or do, they might consider it to be mischievous in nature when in fact it is coming from the innocence of a 5 year old in a man's body. It's not bad. It just sounds that way, if you don't know the difference and don't know how I think. Depending on the mindset of the person, what I say might raise eyebrows with one person thinking I just said or asked the most horrible thing on earth and another person might hear me say the same thing or ask the same thing and think, "Oh, how cute. You're such a sweetie. Sure I can do that." Or, "So, is this what you're saying? That's fine. No problem." That's the reason I left the remainder of the things I wanted to tell you about me out of here because I didn't want to take chances on what few nurses that couldn't possibly understand getting a hold of this book and thinking, "Just who do you think you are?" when I didn't even mean anything bad by anything to begin with.

## To Nurse Means To Nurture: Part Two

Like I said, not all nurses would feel that way about the things I'm telling you about, just some of them would. It would just be a disaster if someone that did not understand made a big deal out of the whole thing and wanted to put me in my place because they think I'm horrible. Just because it's different doesn't mean it's bad. Remember this when you are taking care of those with disabled people suffering from Autism and show them all the love and care you can.

Most autistics don't like touch like I do so they have to be dealt differently from me but autistics like myself who crave touch need to be showed all the love and affection and hugs you can possibly show them and feel accepted by and cared for by you no matter what they say or do that makes you feel weird. Be willing to forgive them and go on and don't let it bother you. They are the way they are because that's the way they are and you as a nurse are like a parent to them because the nurse-patient relationship is really that of a "mother and child" relationship in the medical setting. Thank you for your understanding and compassion and love. Please show your patients you love them, especially the disabled, and care for them as if they were your own little child. They need you and they need your love. Please be there for them. This is one of the best things you could do for anybody when you do this.

## To Nurse Means to Nurture Part Two
## The Parent Role of the Nurse with All Ages of Patients

Hi everybody. I was hoping you had a new concept about what a nurse is and what it means to be a nurse and what being a nurse entails from a compassionate standpoint from reading my other book. I would now like to take this a step further to show you even more proof of the same thing that shows your role as a nurse being the "surrogate mother" of your patients and show you just how that plays into the whole circle of things by showing you even more book references or any other references I might find that show all this.

The following are quotes concerning how nurses handle both the ideal patient to them and how they handle someone who is difficult for them to deal with or they may even find annoying. I found these in "Basic Nursing, A Psychophysiologic Approach, page 132"."

"A nurse's moods and behaviors may actually increase suffering of some patients physically as well as psychologically and may delay their recovery."
> Basic Nursing: A Psychophysiologic Approach, Sorenson Luckmann, W.B. Saunders Company, 1979, page 132

When you as a nurse are in a bad mood or show contempt for a certain patient or you act harshly with them it can hurt them emotionally and make them feel like they are being scolded or punished for things you don't like that they said or did that might not have crossed you the right way, or they said something stupid or childish you may have took the wrong way and made something out of it that really wasn't there they feel like a nuisance, a failure, and a low down piece of dirt, or an ant in your presence, and feel like they are at your mercy.

They technically already feel like they are at your mercy to some extent just being your patient, but when you treat them harshly or lecture them sternly or even punish them for things that annoy you they really feel like they are at your mercy then.

## To Nurse Means To Nurture: Part Two

They feel like they have to walk on egg shells to say anything to you of any sort from then on because they are afraid they will say the wrong thing and they are afraid of how you will react and may be worried sick you will jump down their throat if they say the wrong thing. I have run into this situation myself several times before. I usually run into this with people that don't understand me to begin with, but because I do say some stupid things and do some stupid things sometimes there are times when even nice nurses might want to let me have it because they can't believe I could be so stupid because I say stupid things some times or make a wrong decision about something. That usually doesn't happen with a nice, chipper acting female nurse, though, but when it does happen I feel like I've really failed then and messed up everything because I feel like the only nurse that may understand me may be offended by what I said and never let me hear the end of it or things may never be the same again and I may lose a friend. Sometimes I may even say things that embarrass them or me or both of us. I've said stupid things to people in public before not thinking before I spoke and made them blush before and I would wind up apologizing all over the place about it and saying, "I'm sorry. I didn't mean to embarrass you. I shouldn't have said that." I worry that my needs my never be met again by whoever the nurse is if they are meeting them or they will be forever be upset with me and hold a grudge. I have autism and because of my autism sometimes I say things or ask things of people that may sound a little too personal for their comfort. When I say things like this or ask things like this I mean nothing amiss but my fear is that they won't know that and they will think I mean something amiss. It all depends on the interpreter of the statements I make and the questions I ask. One nurse if I say something or ask something that sounds odd they might think, "Ah…That's really cute." or "You're sweet."

With another nurse I could say the exact same thing or ask the exact same question to them and they might jump down my throat and say, "No I can't do this!" in an angry tone of voice if it's a question or "How could you say such a stupid thing? What's the matter with you? Have you totally lost your mind?" in an angry tone of voice and act very stern with me when they say it.

There are some times that I worry my self sick over things I say to nurses after I say them thinking, "Oh no. They're probably not going to like me anymore after I said this or asked that. They're probably going to hate me forever. Now I've really blown it. They'll never trust me again or meet my needs again because they think I mean something horrible by whatever I just said when whatever I came up with was just nothing but a stupid statement or a stupid question I didn't have the brains not to say or ask." The thing is there have been some times I lived in fear all the way to the next appointment after I did something like this, thinking "What if? What if?" thinking it was all about to come to an end, and I might go to my next appointment and find out the nurse was never even offended with me to begin with. So, when I go to the next appointment about to shrivel up in fear thinking, "I've really done it now. They're going to hate me for sure now." They may say, "Is something wrong? What is it your worried about? Is something bothering you?" I might say, "I said this or I said that or I asked you this or that and I didn't mean anything bad by it but I thought you would take me wrong for saying whatever it was and hate me forever and never meet my needs again." And, then that very nurse says, "Is that what you were worried about? I'm sorry. I didn't mean for you to have to worry your self sick for the next two or three weeks just because you thought you said or did something wrong. I wasn't offended at all. You didn't do anything wrong. As a matter of fact, I think what you said was cute." Or, "I thought it was neat that you asked me that. That was sweet. Don't worry about that. I'm not offended at all. You worried all this time all for nothing and everything's the same as it always was. Everything's okay. You're just fine. I didn't think a thing wrong of what you said or asked." Yet, you may think because this is the kind of nurse that will probably think something is cute or sweet they probably won't jump down your throat for it but you're not sure because other disgruntled nurses out there may have jumped down your throat before for saying the same thing or something similar to it and you think, "I'd hate to be wrong. I don't want to lose my favorite nurse. I'll never be able to have the kind of thing going with a nurse like this again. I've waited a long time for someone to understand me like they do and now I've ruined everything."

## To Nurse Means To Nurture: Part Two

This is very traumatic for me when this happens. When this happens I feel like all hope is gone. Luckily, it's not normally someone I already like this happens with but sometimes it is, and that's even worse than when it is not. I just want to be able to be myself and be allowed to say or ask some of the childlike things I say or ask you may not have yet heard me say or ask without feeling like I have to walk on egg shells and be able to say these things when I think of them without being judged. I just want you to be willing to respond to me like you would a kid if they said or asked you the same things I do when I come up with these things.

Have any of you ever heard about how Peter the disciple in the Bible always seemed to say the wrong things at the first? I'm not trying to make myself equal with Peter because the kinds of things I say to people that are stupid are far worse than anything he would come up with, but just as Peter says stupid things and doesn't mean anything amiss by anything he says, neither do I mean anything amiss when I say the wrong things and mess it up for myself.

I don't know if you remember this or not, but when the disciple Peter did mess up, Jesus didn't come down hard on him and act harshly with him, he just nicely corrected him in a round about way that he could understand in order to get him to see what he said wrong without hurting his feelings. He didn't lecture him for it all over the place and make him feel miserable for it because he knew Peter meant nothing bad by what he said, he just tried to get Peter to see in a nice way, and why what he said was wrong. So, if I ever do this to you, please don't deal with me harshly if I offend you but talk to me the way Jesus talked to Peter to state your feelings on the issue but try not to say it in a condescending way. I know I sometimes say stupid things before I think, but please forgive me when I do this because I mean nothing by it when I do.

Now, as far as my list of needs go, that may sound strange to you too, but that I have to have met a certain way no matter how weird it makes you feel.

I have to be able to get hugs from all my nurses and get all "chipper acting, cheery" female nurses only and no "males or "serious trended" females for nurses and they have to be willing to rub my head to calm me down and hold my hand through needle sticks and be willing to show me lots of affection and attention and be patient with me and treat me like a mother would treat their own children because of my childlike needs. That I can't change. That all has to stay the same.

But, if I say something that does not apply to this list of needs that is just plain silly and that offends you, please just be willing to blow it off and say to yourself, "He's just being a kid. He doesn't mean anything by it. Leave him be." And, if it really bugs you and gets on your nerves please just try to be nice about telling me and not come down hard on me and forgive me for saying whatever it is, just make sure you meet my needs and don't condemn me for asking you to meet my needs. Thank you. I really appreciate your understanding. Please read even further all the rest of the comments I have here as it expresses my feelings and emotions and how I need you to be with me and practically takes the words right out of my mouth even though it came out of a college textbook of nursing.

"What behavioral qualities might patients find helpful in a nurse? Frequently people who are ill want to be "cared for" by a person who is "accepting", "thoughtful", "gentle", "nurturing", "kind", "genuine", "emotionally warm", "caring" and "giving".
    Basic Nursing: A Psychophysiologic Approach, Sorenson Luckmann, W.B. Saunders Company, 1979, page 132

"At times a nurse may feel a sense of discomfort in response to what a patient is saying or the specific manner in which he is acting, however, she still strives to convey a genuine acceptance of the patient as a person. That is to say, the attitude the nurse tries to convey to the patient is: "I care about you even though these particular words or this specific behavior of yours makes me uncomfortable."
    Basic Nursing: A Psychophysiologic Approach, Sorenson Luckmann, W.B. Saunders Company, 1979, page 132

I need you to care for me no matter what I say or do.

This acceptance of the patient as a person requires that the nurse demonstrate a genuine appreciation of the patient's situation rather than only looking at this behavior by itself and reacting to it without attempting to understand what prompts the behavior."
    Basic Nursing, A Psychophysiologic Approach, Sorenson Luckmann, W.B. Saunders Company, 1979, Page 132

"The hallmark of a truly professional nurse is not merely her ability to take care of patients whom she personally likes and whose pleasant moods and behaviors make her feel good. The professional nurse has the ability to also care for, and about, those patients (often called "difficult") whom she may find personally upsetting. Such a nurse does not expect everyone to be of a similar disposition or even that a given individual will be consistently pleasant, nor does she expect other people to be consistently attune their moods to hers. A sensitive nurse is adaptable to patients' moods. She learns to sense when levity might be enjoyed, for example, and when it is out of place, when patients need to be alone as well as when her presence can be helpful."
    Basic Nursing, A Psychophysiologic Approach, Sorenson Luckmann, W.B. Saunders Company, 1979, Page 133

"Patients who feel they cannot trust us are frightened and justly so, for they often place their life in our hands. In such a situation, it is most important to let the person talk about what happened in the past and to remain nonjudgmental yet supportive."
    Basic Nursing: A Psychophysiologic Approach, Sorenson Luckmann, W.B. Saunders Company, 1979, page 142

I have felt like I had trouble trusting nurses my whole life because of all my bad experiences I had with them throughout my lifetime and especially during the timeframe of Birth through Junior High when my absolute worst experiences with male doctors, male nurses, and serious trended female nurses occurred. That's more from a standpoint of what they will do to me physically and verbally in the process.

## To Nurse Means To Nurture: Part Two

Several serious trended female nurses during my adulthood also tortured me with needles and acted rude to me. As a matter of fact, I feel like I have to be afraid of telling new doctors and nurses what happened to me in the past at the military hospital I went to from Birth to Age 21 and the institute I was in from Age 13 to 14 ½ for being wild as a child because of things these people did that were graphic in nature because I might be judged for being inappropriate when I'm actually telling the truth. The stories of what these people did to me are in Chapter One and Chapter Three of "Big City Hospitals Don't Like Cowards". This would be in my most revised copy of it. The one in Chapter One has a Part II and Part III in later chapters in the first part of that book. As far as the chipper acting female nurses during adulthood, most of them have done very well with me, understood me very well, and met all my needs very well, and comforted me the way I asked them to, and tried to calm my fears when I was scared and showed me plenty of affection when they did.

However, in the past couple of years, I've suddenly run into nurses, even chipper acting females who suddenly decided it was not in their job description to comfort their patients and that I was in the wrong for daring to even ask assuming I must have horrible intentions for even asking for them and asking them to do what I need them to do for me, when they are the kinds of nurses that always were there for me in the past and comforted me by giving me hugs and rubbing my head to calm me down and holding my hand through needle sticks. What got into some of these people I don't know? Most of the ones that came up with this were all "new nurses" I never met before that had a totally different concept of nursing than all the other chipper acting female nurses that took care of me in the past that met all my needs willingly and happily. That's why I wrote my last book, "To Nurse Means to Nurture: The Need for Nurses to Comfort their Patients" to show that it is in fact in their job description to comfort their patients whether they believe it to be so or not and yes, that does include touching.

## To Nurse Means To Nurture: Part Two

I have a fear that they will be impersonal all because they decided it is not in their job description to comfort their patients and think they are supposed to go around acting like "stoic" mechanics fixing a bunch of machines instead of treating the patient like a person and meeting their emotional needs and being like a mother to them. If they went back and reread some of their own books they would see that for themselves considering that is where I am getting most of my information on the subject from, their books.

In this book, not only would I like to show you as I did earlier in the first book that the nurse is the "mother surrogate" of the patient, but the whole team of nurses is a "surrogate family" to the patient. You think I'm joking. Keep reading. I'm about to show you where I got this from in the next few quotes.

"General state of personal happiness: persons who are happy and feel loved may find illness and hospitalization difficult to bear because it means separation from home and loved ones; on the other hand, lonely unhappy people may feel they receive more attention, and are the object of more concern when ill than when they are well."
    Basic Nursing: A Psychophysiologic Approach, Sorenson Luckmann, W.B. Saunders Company, 1979, page 148

I've felt both ways before because there have been some hospital situations that were so horrible to me that it was difficult to bear. However, in a hospital setting where all my needs are met I do feel like I receive more attention and am the object of more concern when ill than when well because outside of the hospital I sometimes feel like a fish out of water because I am different in various ways that count me out in my normal everyday life.
I like to hang out more with ladies than men. I have the interests of ladies and little kids. I feel out of place with men that are all into hunting and automobile mechanics and electronics and plumbing and the like. I'm not into sports either. I am more into kid movies, board games, Christmas trinkets, antique girl dolls, quilts, coloring books, walking trails, taking pictures with a digital camera and enhancing them on the computer and then printing off cards and calendars with them.

I also like painting, growing a flower garden, having tea parties with other ladies, having Birthday parties and Christmas parties etc. Because of this I feel almost left out or out of place, because even though there are ladies that are more than willing to do this with me, I feel like the opportunities I get to have this kind of fun with other ladies like the tea parties and picnics and such are far and in between. Most of this stuff they like to do together is done at ladies' events and I get left out in the process. Plus, there's not a lot of people that interested in watching kid movies and playing board games with me and they really feel like they don't want to have to babysit me because they feel like their having to take care of a 5-year-old when they are around me and really don't want bothered with it. And, even if these events come up that I am invited to I'm too tired half the time to go to them or get overtired if I have to do them for too long.

Don't get the wrong idea though, some people may look at this and think I must be gay to have all these kinds of interests. Actually I am far from gay and the type of thinking these people have is far from my mind. I'm a ladies' guy and I've met people like this before who were not gay, but they just like to hang around the ladies because that was just their preference. I had all this when I was in Special Ed and I lost all that when I got out of Special Ed. There was a guy I knew once that owned a beauty shop I went to when my mother went to get her hair done there when I was a kid. This guy still owned this place up to about a couple of years ago before he died. That's what he was comfortable with, because like me, guys were just too rough house for him and he just flat don't have the same interests as them. He surrounded himself with mostly women and only occasionally had a guy come in he talked to. He really enjoyed his environment and the company of the women he was with. That was just his preference because that was just the way he was and that was his personality. I really liked this guy a lot since childhood and this guy liked me too. I thought the guy was really neat. That's the way I am too and that's the way I like it. I was friends with this guy at the beauty shop when I went there to wait for my mother to get her hair done.

I talked to him some of the time and made friends with him but I spent most of my time visiting with the other lady beauticians or reading magazines while I waited for my mother to get done because like him, I still liked being with the ladies better. Most guys are not artsy entertainment types. Most guys are macho or tough acting or competition driven or like sports. I like competition too but I like it with art and music and not race car driving if you know what I mean. I'm not into sports either. I'm just an artsy entertainment guy who also likes to take pictures and paint and shop in gift shops, watch kid movies, color in color books, walk trials, go on picnics, listen to Christmas records and Christmas movies, have Christmas Parties and Birthday parties and Tea Parties and the like. I'm quite different from other guys you see. And, I am a much more emotional person than other guys are. I tend to be moved by things like other women would be that other guys are too rough house or too macho to even think about being moved about.

So, if you ever put me in a home, please do not stick me in a place with a whole bunch of guys because I'm a guy or give me a guy nurse or guy aide because I am a guy because I feel out of place with these people and it depresses me when I am thrown off on guys when girls are the ones I am comfortable with and relate to. I for sure don't want male nurses. I don't even want them to give me a bath if I'm in a hospital or nursing home. I want a chipper acting female nurse to do it. Besides that, I would feel weird having a guy bathe me even if I was okay with them. I'm not okay with it because I need the motherly personality of a chipper acting female nurse to take care of all my needs including giving me a bath and toileting if that particular scenario ever comes up where I have to be bathed or toileted by a nurse due to inability to perform normal functions of daily living that I can perform myself now. I really don't like male nurses and don't want them either. When "male" doctors and "male" nurses and "serious trended" female nurses see me naked I feel like a peon slave they wish to torture. When a chipper acting female nurse sees me naked I feel like a baby in diapers. I also feel safer this way.

I'm not trying to be inappropriate by making this statement. I'm just trying to point out that the attitude "males" and "serious trended" female nurses had toward me when they got me undressed in front of them was "Try to stop me now, you peon slave!" and every time a "chipper acting" female nurse even made me get undressed in front of them their attitude was, "He's just a sweet little baby in diapers and I'm just taking care of him like I was his own mother."

"Male" nurses tortured me as a kid, as well as "male" doctors. And many now even act mean and gruff, as they did then.

I need the comfort of a "motherly female nurse" who babies me to death and shows me lots of "love and affection" and gives me lots of "hugs" and "comforts me through all my needle sticks and other scary procedures."

I know you guys are probably thinking, "Give me a break. I'm not your mother. Do you have to be so needy with me?" but actually you are, you're my "mother surrogate" and you are about to find out you're all my "mother surrogates".

Keep reading for more quotes from one of your own books. Here it comes.

"Patients who are suspicious are not just complaining; they are frightened and feel that they must be on their guard or they will be hurt or taken advantage of."
    Basic Nursing: A Psychophysiologic Approach, Sorenson Luckmann, W.B. Saunders Company, 1979, page 151

Like my fears of this happening because "male" doctors, 'male" nurses, and "serious trended" female nurses all did this to me as a kid and then "serious trended" female nurses continued to be this way with me clear into adulthood and beyond. That's why I insist on "chipper acting, cheery" female nurses because they are "motherly" and "compassionate" and "sweet" and "fun loving" and "adventurous" and "playful" and "comforting" and "consoling" in their character.

To Nurse Means To Nurture: Part Two

"The specific fears that accompany the realization that one has a dreaded illness are many. Here is a list of some specific fears that accompany illness:

1. Fear of a strange place, e.g., the hospital, nursing home, and so forth
2. Fear of equipment – "Will it hurt me? What is if doesn't run right?"
3. Fear of pain, loss of body parts, or mutilation
4. Fear of being "experimented on"
5. Fear of having to suffer as punishment for past behavior
6. Fear or treatments and diagnostic processes, e.g., surgery, cardiac catherizations
7. Fear of being abused or neglected; of having one's feelings hurt, or being "treated impersonally."
8. Fear of being "left alone" or "isolated from loved ones"
9. Fear of loss of function or loss of self-control
10. Fear of death
11. Fear of "burdening others"

Basic Nursing: A Psychophysiologic Approach, Sorenson Luckmann, W.B. Saunders Company, 1979, page 152 & 153

My top fear is that of being neglected, having my feelings hurt or being treated impersonal by a nurse.

My other main fears are being in a strange place, being afraid the equipment will hurt me, especially needles and scalpels and anything else sharp, being punished for behaviors a nurse might not like because they don't understand my autism, my fear of diagnostic procedures such as surgery and cardiac catherizations, how much they will hurt and whether the nurses will comfort me the way I want comforted and need comforted or that I will get the kind of nurses I want and need, chipper acting female nurses only, fear of being left alone or isolated from others, and becoming a burden to those nurses taking care of me and being scolded for saying or doing things they may not understand or the fact they think I am bugging them too much and wish I would just leave them alone.

I really need a lot of attention and affection and I need nurses to be patient with me each time they see me and throughout any hospital stays I may have no matter how big a burden I may be to them.

"In illness it should be expected that patients will regress to levels of behavior that are not as mature as those which they assume when well. They need to be allowed sufficient and appropriate regression and dependence in others."
>Basic Nursing: A Psychophysiologic Approach, Sorenson Luckmann, W.B. Saunders Company, 1979, page 152

"Ill persons have a strong 'need' for security, 'warm', 'friendly' interactions and familiar settings promote feelings of security."
>Basic Nursing: A Psychophysiologic Approach, Sorenson Luckmann, W.B. Saunders Company, 1979, page 15

>I have a dire need for warm, friendly interactions from my nurses and I have a dire need to receive chipper acting, cheery female nurses only to show me motherly love and care and provide a great deal of attention and affection for me, be willing to give me lots of hugs (let me press my right ear on their cheek), and rub my head to calm me down and hold my hand through needle sticks such as blood tests, IVs, shots, biopsies, tubes of any kind, blades, scalpels, or anything else sharp. I need to be able to put Lidocaine/Prilocaine 2.5% cream on the site of the stick before you stick me with needles and I need put completely put to sleep for all invasive procedures. No males and no serious trended females for nurses, techs, or anesthesiologist, or any other medical professional. Chipper acting, cheery female nurses only who will comfort and console me in all my fear and pain and stay with me and be present for me and show compassion toward me. This is very important to me and this is what I need. I cannot have it any other way. Only this will work.

"Emotional regression (going back to earlier stages of psychological development) may produce conflict for a patient if he realizes that although he is an adult, and thus should act as an adult, he 'wants to' or 'needs' to act in a rather 'childlike ways'".
> Basic Nursing: A Psychophysiologic Approach, Sorenson Luckmann, W.B. Saunders Company, 1979, page 152

I need to be able to open up and be able to act like a child and be treated like a child and be allowed to say childish things and make childish requests when I am with nurses especially in the hospital setting and I need to be able to comforted like a child because I have childlike needs. If I say something stupid at any point that a nurse might normally take wrong, I need them to look at it like, "He's just being a kid. Don't be down on him. He's just a child in a man's body acting like a child because he's socially and emotionally 5 years old whether he's an adult or not so let him be that way and don't make anything of it. He's just being a kid.

Besides that he requires a lot of attention and affection because of his disability and he needs us to be like mothers to him. If he says anything strange don't take it too seriously, he's just being a kid at heart. He doesn't mean anything by it. And, if he asks us to baby him to death, just do it, he wants us to be his mothers and this is what he needs."

"In their search for security patients often hope to find in nurses the reassuring qualities of sympathy, tenderness, understanding, and gentleness tempered with firmness. The careful reader will observe that these are qualities often attributed in the "ideal mother figure."
> Basic Nursing: A Psychophysiologic Approach, Sorenson Luckmann, W.B. Saunders Company, 1979, page 152

"The patient thus often looks to his doctors and nurses for protection from life's adversities. The regressed patient, seeking these qualities of ideal parents in staff members is disappointed by the absence of such qualities. Thoughtful health professionals strive to enhance patients' feelings of security and warmth by helping make the environment (shared by both staff and patients) as comfortable and as warm as possible."
      Basic Nursing: A Psychophysiologic Approach, Sorenson Luckmann, W.B. Saunders Company, 1979, page 152

I need chipper acting, cheery female nurses only and I need them all to give me hugs and rub my head to calm me down and hold my hand through blood tests, shots, IVs, biopsies, or any other experiences involving sharp instruments just like I said in my first book I wrote about nurses comforting their patients.

"For some patients, e.g. patients in long term health care facilities, staff members become "pseudo-family members." These patients (and others) look to the staff for "protection", "warmth", "guidance", "support", "modeling", expectations and judgment they would hope to receive from their family. Security is enhanced for patients' expectations of them. It is thus desirable for health professionals to assess a patient's expectations of them and to identify ways in which these expectations can be dealt with constructively."
      Basic Nursing: A Psychophysiologic Approach, Sorenson Luckmann, W.B. Saunders Company, 1979, page 152

Like I said, some nurses I've run into in the past may think, "He acts like such a baby. Why do we have to deal with this? Why doesn't he just grow up? Do we have to baby him to death all the time and always do all these special things for him? Why do we have to be stuck with having to do this anyway?" And, as you can see here, the answer is, "Well, you may feel that way, and like some have said, they feel like taking care of me is like having to take care of a kindergartner and they really don't like it, but if you really think about it, that's what you're there for because you are the nurses and you are the "mother surrogates" of all your patients.

## To Nurse Means To Nurture: Part Two

This is especially true for disabled patients with special needs like my self and this is really what you need to do to make life better for both your patients and yourselves, and all goes better in the end when you do.

"Persons who receive their care from the same health practitioner are more compliant than those who are treated or examined by different practitioners. The explanation may be a combination of interpersonal "comfort", "ease of communication", and a "saving in time needed to explain problems".
>Comprehensive Rehabilitation Nursing, Nancy Martin, Nancye B. Holt, Dorothy Hicks, McGraw Hill Book Company, 1981, page 60

I do more for my nurse practitioner because she comforts me when I need her to and so does her daughter. She is very good to me, takes out time to listen to me, and advocates for me to others to help them understand my needs like she understands my needs.

"The brevity of the usual patient record also detracts from the ease with which another practitioner takes over. Problem-oriented records and flow sheets stating physical findings, lab tests, and medications or treatments are helpful in allowing a practitioner new to the case to grasp the whole picture. These records also assist the person's usual caregiver in following progress."
>Comprehensive Rehabilitation Nursing, Nancy Martin, Nancye B. Holt, Dorothy Hicks, McGraw Hill Book Company, 1981, page 60

"The relationship between the patient and the health practitioner is one of the more important factors in compliance. This factor is difficult to measure, but that is probably not the reason few studies focus on it as a variable in compliance. The current emphasis on "patient characteristics" is a probable reason. Studies dealing with the relationship have examined it from the standpoint of patterns and content of communication on the part of the practitioner (usually the physician), "patient satisfaction with the encounter", "extent to which patient expectations are met", "amount of reciprocal interaction between patient and practitioner", and "congruity between what the patient thinks he or she is to do and what the practitioner thinks the patient is doing." In general, the studies have indicated that when the practitioner communicates in a formal, controlling manner, when there is little reciprocal interaction, and when patients' expectations are unmet, compliance is low."
>Comprehensive Rehabilitation Nursing, Nancy Martin, Nancye B. Holt, Dorothy Hicks, McGraw Hill Book Company, 1981, page 60

If my family doctor nurse practitioner is reading this please do not be alarmed by the second half of this quote because you have never acted this way toward me.

I do have to say though because of my anxiety and fears not knowing what to expect, that if I ever said anything to offend you that regardless of you never having acted this way toward me ever before you might begin to act this way toward me if I offended you and if you did I would feel hopeless forever and feel like I just lost my best friend.

Other nurses or doctors, if I ever offended them all I would have to do is say one thing wrong or do one thing wrong they didn't like and they wound up treating me like they hated me ever since. If I did offend one it was usually something trivial or they just never understood my emotional needs in the first place. Thank you so much for understanding me. Please don't ever turn the other way.

So, please, if I ever say anything to offend you, no matter what it is I said, even if you think what I said is too personal or you think I somehow said something out of line and it has upset you, please, I beg you to forgive me and never hold it against me and always be the same as you always have been. I'm sorry if I ever said anything wrong, and if I haven't said anything wrong I'm sorry if I ever do say anything wrong because I am autistic and sometimes can't always help what I say or speak before I think, and it's usually not anything mean or anything, its usually something you would probably think was sweet or cute, but not being certain of the reaction to what I might say if it was taken wrong, I live in fear of anything I might say that might ever offend you and it would traumatize me tremendously if I ever said the wrong thing and turned you away from me, so please don't let things like this stop you from continuing to be my friend and continuing to meet my needs because I could not handle it if it ever fell apart. I waited too long to get it this good to mess things up and I don't want to mess it up now, so please forgive me if I ever do because it is completely unintentional. Thank you.

I have run into other nurses before that have acted this way toward me before, especially if they have a "serious trended" personality.

The ones with the "serious acting personalities" have the tendency to see me as a "piece of property" which they can run over like a doormat and it is in a controlling manner they do this because their attitude is obey me or else. For situations I have had at hospitals like the one I had 12 years ago and like the one I had at the military hospital the first 21 years of my life where doctors and nurses want to use absolute force to control a patient's every move, especially someone with a disability they consider to be a nuisance and a troublemaker to them and do everything they can to detain them in a hospital setting and never let them go as best as they can, I found the following statement in a college textbook of nursing these people of this nature may find shocking that insist on being this way.

"False imprisonment consists of unjustifiably restraining another person by force or threats of force. It may be a problem for the nurse in two situations. The first arises when a patient wants to leave the hospital and the hospital does not want him to leave, either because his physician advises that he should remain hospitalized or because he has not paid his bill. In neither case may he legally be detained by force or threats of force. In the former case, he is customarily asked to sign a statement that he is leaving against medical advice and absolving the hospital of liability for damages caused by his early departure. But he cannot be detained even if he refuses to sign such as statement. And in the latter case, the hospital does not have even an arguable claim to detain him. Telling him that he cannot leave the hospital might, under the circumstances, be construed as a threat of force and is hence risky. The other situation concerns the application of restraints. If use of restraints is reasonably necessary to protect the patient or others it is justifiable and hence not false imprisonment. At the same time, failure to use restraints when they are required is negligence. But any unnecessary use of restraints constitutes false imprisonment. Application of restraints directly to the patient's body will also amount to batter unless there is justification."
 Basic Nursing: A Psychophysiologic Approach, Sorensen, Luckmann, W. B. Saunders Company, 1979, page

"The more nurses know and understand about brain-damaged patients, the more efficient they will be as observers. Early writings on brain-damaged individuals frequently stated that such patients demonstrated catastrophic behavior. When the behavior was analyzed, its cause was more frequently the interaction between the health practitioner and the patient than organic conditions. A lack of understanding by nurses of brain-damaged patients and their learning functioning often affects patients' total adjustment and their eventual rehabilitation accomplishments. The individuality and the particular problems of each patient must be understood by the health practitioner if the patient is to succeed in any rehabilitation program. Again, the nurse who is in constant contact with patients is the one with the best opportunity to achieve this understanding."

> Comprehensive Rehabilitation Nursing, Nancy Martin, Nancye B. Holt, Dorothy Hicks, McGraw Hill Book Company, 1981, page 137

"Whether brain damage has resulted from trauma or from a stroke, the patients previously functioned in a variety of ways with a variety of skills which may or may not be available to them now. The nurse attempts to relate medical findings on a patient to the cognitive functions that the patient demonstrates. To do this, it is necessary to understand all the processes by which the patient receives sensory input and how that sensory input is transferred, reduced, elaborated, stated, recovered, and eventually used for life and living. The brain-injured individual is a complicated individual."

> Comprehensive Rehabilitation Nursing, Nancy Martin, Nancye B. Holt, Dorothy Hicks, McGraw Hill Book Company, 1981, page 137

"Another key word to understanding is individuality. Although clinicians attempt to categorize disabilities and understand the psychology of each disability, nurses cannot lose track of the unique aspects of each human being and the unique skills, past learning experiences, environmental, social, and family influences that have mad that individual."

> Comprehensive Rehabilitation Nursing, Nancy Martin, Nancye B. Holt, Dorothy Hicks, McGraw Hill Book Company, 1981, page 137

I do have brain damage, but my brain damage is not from a brain injury rather it is from turning blue at birth and a result of autism. There are things that are different about me that some people may find hard to understand. I may not be interested in the same things the typical guy is interested in or even the normal everyday person for that matter. I am more interested in things of both a girlish nature and a kid like nature. Even the thoughts I have about things that may be misunderstood by other individuals when I express them may not be the most common thinking of the average individual. Most of the thoughts I have that are taken wrong are actually more like that of a kid than that of an adult.

As a matter of fact, I may not even be affected the same way by certain things that other individuals are affected by. There are things that affect me from a childlike standpoint in some instances where I may want or like a certain thing or need a certain thing because I am actually affected the same way as a child would be affected by the same thing or another Special Ed person rather than that of the normal everyday individual. I may have totally innocent motives for things I like, want, or ask for and some normal person that would want or ask for the same things might have totally different motives of a horrible nature. There have been things I asked people in the past that I meant nothing amiss about at all and then I was eventually shocked to find out from someone else that if someone else made the same request they would have bad intentions. Nurses need to keep this in mind if I say something odd or ask something odd because what they may perceive as horrible may be nothing more than a childish autistic quirk I have that I have a hang-up about or something that bugs the life out of me that I feel like I've just got to resolve before it drives me crazy.

I found this comment in a book about meeting the special needs of an autistic person, possibly even needs that may seem strange to you in a book another individual wrote on Autism in Healthcare:

"If the person with autism doesn't understand what is involved in surgery, where do practitioners begin to communicate what is to happen? One ground-breaking study reported in the journal Pediatric Anesthesia demonstrates the great success of a management program specifically designed to enable children with autism to be admitted for medical and surgical procedures (Van der Walt and Moran 2001).
      Health Care and the Autism Spectrum, A Guide For Health Professionals, Parents and Carers, Alison Morton-Cooper, page 73, Jessica Kingsley Publishers, 2004

"Autism is beginning to explain a good deal of the emotional and behavioral difficulty of people who in the past have been labeled extremely eccentric or rude."
>Health Care and the Autism Spectrum, A Guide For Health Professionals, Parents and Carers, Alison Morton-Cooper, page 46, Jessica Kingsley Publishers, 2004

"Even in the most able people with autism, serious communication deficits may remain, though they may be well hidden behind the characteristic stilted, pedantic, and over-complex language of the more intellectually able person with autism."
>Health Care and the Autism Spectrum, A Guide For Health Professionals, Parents and Carers, Alison Morton-Cooper, page 73, Jessica Kingsley Publishers, 2004

On this next page is a list of things that a program in the Health Care and Autism Book that they suggest a parent or caregiver or guardian give to the nursing staff of the hospital when they take them there. Believe it or not, not only does it tell you to list the autistic person's needs but it also tells you to list their "likes", "dislikes", and "fetishes". So chances are, even the stuff that may embarrass you to know about them is on there.

They can be kind of odd and so can I so you just need to be able to accept them like they are and go on no matter how weird it makes you feel.

"The program was devised because of the great difficulties experienced by clinicians in trying to manage such children using normal procedures. The authors recognized that children with autism are a neglected group with the well-defined needs that have not been adequately considered in the anesthetic literature. They set about rectifying this by setting up a system that identified these children in advance and that alerted anesthetic staff to the fact that the children would be attending for surgery. Management guidelines and specialist pre-admission procedures (including an Autistic Anesthetic Questionnaire) are used to elicit specific responses regarding the nature and severity of the child's autism condition (such as severity; developmental level; "likes/fetishes/dislikes", "phobias for food drink, activities, and objects", "special needs" medication; general health; and social/home circumstances). The admission process is individualized to meet the "specific needs of the patient". An anesthesia plan is drawn up and parents consulted. Decisions are made regarding special admission needs, type of premedication, induction of anesthesia and post-operative strategies, and these are shared with the nurse in charge of the unit admitting the patient."

>Health Care and the Autism Spectrum, A Guide For Health Professionals, Parents and Carers, Alison Morton-Cooper, page 73, Jessica Kingsley Publishers, 2004

There is one nurse at the office of a specialist I go to that if I ever have to have a procedure done is going to fix it where I'll be able to get my hugs and my head rubs and hand holds through needle sticks and get chipper acting female nurses only and be completely put to sleep for the procedure and they are going to talk to the surgery room staff to see if there is anyway they can give me the gas first before the IV because of my oversensitivity to pain.

They said if they insisted on giving me the IV before putting me to sleep they were going to ask "Can you at least give him enough gas before the idea to make him a little woozy and a little numb before you even start the IV even if you do the IV before putting him to sleep? I really appreciated that.

To Nurse Means To Nurture: Part Two

I didn't have to have a procedure after all yet, but there for a while it was looking like I would. So far, so good now, but if I ever do have to have one done they have me covered.

They were also going to ask that they give me a female anesthesiologist instead of a male and make sure not to give me any male nurses or serious trended female nurses, but chipper acting, cheery female nurses only who will meet every need I ask them to meet for me. And, if there was not a female anesthesiologist available they were going to ask the male anesthesiologist to stay out of sight and give instructions to a female nurse on what to put in the IV and how to administer it to me so I wouldn't even have to see them. They have that covered too. That's the best service I've had in years.

Here is another quote I found from this book on Health Care and Autism:

"Parents have been labeled as difficult and obstructive for trying to explain why precautions may have to be put in place. Where such advice has been ignored or dismissed, not only do the people involved feel devalued, but the quality of care is put at risk, with the added possibility that behavioral reactions can lead to a loss of control. The main ingredient in any unwanted reaction is likely to be fear and anxiety. By planning to reduce that anxiety the chances of a successful consultation are far greater.

There are several very practical things that the doctor or health professional being consulted can do to minimize risk. These include:

Asking parents/carers or the person concerned to devise a sensory profile of your patient so that you can minimize and address any sensory triggers.

Making appointments at a time when the clinic is relatively quiet (over lunch, at the very beginning or end of the day)

Explaining who you are and what you have been asked to do.

Making sure your patient isn't hungry or over-tired.

Using any special interests your patient may have to help them feel at ease (these include obsessive interests of all sorts from ants to train timetables, fascination with numbers, or a special toy).

Recognizing when you are beginning to get into difficulty (being sensitive to small physiological changes that can herald a problem, such as signs of general agitation, increase in heart rate and respiration, flaring of nostrils, grunting, rocking, and pacing).

It is, of course, always important to listen carefully to what patients themselves "say". If they are able to communicate clearly through language, examine their behavior as a communicative act – if the behavior could speak what would it say?"
> Health Care and the Autism Spectrum, A Guide For Health Professionals, Parents and Carers, Alison Morton-Cooper, Jessica Kingsley Publishers, 2004, page 55

I'm actually adult with autism and not a kid with autism but I am like a child sociably and emotionally although near normal for an adult in the area of school work and I still have sensory issues that have to be dealt with and always will. People have to be willing to do what I need them to do to tame these sensory issues like putting my right ear on their cheek to soothe my ear from the stimuli it has that can only be relieved by pressing in on another person's cheek. Also, things like putting Lidocaine/Prilocaine 2.5% cream on one hour before a needle stick at the site of the stick to help relieve my oversensitivity to pain.

My need for comfort and affection has to be met by chipper acting female nurses only who have motherly personalities and steer clear away from giving me any male nurses or serious trended female nurses because I am afraid of them. Both tortured me as a child and the serious trended female nurses also tortured me into adulthood. I need the motherly love a chipper acting cheery female nurse to treat me as if I was their own little baby boy. It sounds crazy, but because of my autism, this is what I need.

And, if you remember, I had a quote earlier that says that nurse need to be willing to let their patients regress and act as a child in childlike ways and be able to make childlike requests to their nurses and actually have them met because this is what they need.

Some other weird things I have about me I noticed that I read about in a book that fit my situation are my problem with certain "fears" that may not make sense to anyone else either. This is associated with my autism too.

"Autistic children also exhibit strange fears – usually of totally harmless objects such as a "bush" or a box, but do not register fear when there is real danger. This is probably connected to their inability to make sense of the impressions they receive."
      Funk & Wagnalls New Encyclopedia of Illustrated Family Health, Marshall Cavendish Limited, 1988, page 108

I had a fear of a bush when I was a kid. I was always afraid of the dark and still am. I'm afraid of fast moving objects or driving fast. I have a fear of heights. I have a fear of storms. I have a fear of needles. I have a fear of snakes. I have a fear of rejection. I have a fear of abandonment. I have a fear of being misunderstood.

Some autistic people seem normal but are actually quite immature in certain ways which you usually will not be able to see right away until you get around them a while. They may have odd thoughts or do odd things or not get it about things you thought sure they would be able to figure out.

"These islands of normality have even led parents of young autistic children to believe that they have had an exceptionally gifted child, putting all other oddities of behavior down to the quirks of genius, until the increasing number of 'quirks" eventually disillusioned them. Such children, who seem to stand astride the dividing line between normality and abnormality, if such a line exists, are sometimes able to live in ordinary society. But they remain immature, vulnerable, and in need of constant support."
      Funk & Wagnalls New Encyclopedia of Illustrated Family Health, Marshall Cavendish Limited, 1988, page 108

This is very true with me as well and I am autistic.

I am vulnerable and I do say and do some things that are immature and I am in constant need of support. I even get confused a lot and don't get things about things other people would get. Sometimes it's the other way around though; sometimes they don't get things I get either. I had a horrible time holding down a job because I couldn't figure out how to do anything right and it aggravated my employers. Plus I wasn't fast enough for them. They always complained, "It took you 6 months to figure out what every one else figured out in one week." And, yes, I may have made some As and Bs in some college classes but only after my mother drilled me to death for hours on end all through junior high and high school until I got it, and still even into my first few years of college. There was always a subject somewhere like Algebra or Music Theory or English Literature or Biology, Physics, or Chemistry that gave me trouble though. I did pretty well in the grammar class but not the literature. I don't get Irony and don't always get jokes people tell. I almost never know what to do in an emergency situation and I can't really cook anything well without messing it up except for bacon, soups, and sandwiches. My meat turns out raw no matter how long I cook it and I can't get recipes to turn out for anything. I may be an adult but you have to remember, I'm disabled. I turned blue at birth and they didn't know I was autistic then and should have listened to my mother when I was 10 years old. My mother tried to tell them she thought I was but they didn't believe it.

A lady diagnosed me with Autism at age 35 years and 10 months old and said it was so obvious that I had it just by looking at my childhood rehab records and by observing me in person in just one hour's time that she thought it was ridiculous these people did not diagnosed me with it back then and they should have known better than that. She said it was obvious and gave me the diagnosis right then and there.

## To Nurse Means To Nurture: Part Two

I think I said earlier I like tea parties, birthday parties, Christmas parties, board games, card games, shopping at gift shops, thrift stores, and antique stores and I like things like quilts, dolls, and pretty stuff.

I even carried a doll to that beauty shop I told you about when I was 12 years old and about embarrassed my mother to death because she thought by that age I should have been over dolls. Plus, I was a guy carrying a girl doll around and that was embarrassing. I used to play with them back then. Now, I just display girl antique dolls on shelves and furniture all over the house along with all my Christmas trinkets.

You've got to keep in mind, I'm not your typical guy and I may appear normal to you and you may think, "What's his problem?" when I come up with something that sounds odd, but I am far from normal, I'm an ex-special Ed student with brain damage that suffers from Autism who turned blue at birth and has special needs that are hard for anyone to understand. I crave touch and require a lot of affection. My entire life I required lots of hugs. I have always needed head rubs and hand holds through needle sticks to comfort me in my fear and pain. I have oversensitivity to pain. A shot feels like a steak knife. A blood test feels like being stabbed with a bigger steak knife. An IV feels like being stabbed with a butcher knife. A catheter feels like a sword being run through me. The way I feel things, the way I perceive things and the way things affect me are totally different from the way every one else is affected.

I constantly worry about what other people think of me and continually fear I will be misunderstood about something and constantly feel like I have to over explain myself about everything just in case one of my friends or nurses or other people happens to interpret something the wrong way.

I may drive you up the wall about something I'm afraid you're going to think about me.

Sometimes I'm afraid to come out and say what it is they think you will take wrong that I said at your office, on the phone, or in a message because they fear the minute they tell you what it is they fear you will take wrong you might jump down their throat and let them have it.

I'm constantly worried you'll take something I say, do, or ask the wrong way. I also have hang-ups about certain things, and I'm always afraid they will be taken wrong too if you know what they are. I'm autistic and that's just the way I am. I mean nothing by it. Once again, I am talking about hang-ups I have I may have said something about or asked you about that don't even have anything to do with my list of needs. If I think you don't understand my list of needs I may worry about that too, but even if something is not on my list of needs, if it's just something I came up with out of the blue that was just driving me up the wall at the moment I told you about I will probably be worried sick about how you took it even if it is a hang-up not associated with my list of needs because I don't want to lose your friendship or be treated differently for it and have to worry about not getting me needs met anymore on account of it. I can be so concerned about this that between office visits if you do not clarify to me that nothing I said has made you upset or the specific thing I thought would make you upset did not make you upset I would worry myself sick about it the entire time until you tell me everything is okay. And sometimes, if I'm really extremely worried about it, I may even fear your reaction to them until they see you to your face a second time and see that all their worries were all for nothing.

Sometimes this can be so overwhelming to me in not knowing how you feel about me that I might be so worked up about it that by the time I finally do go to your office I get the shakes over it and am lucky I don't fall in the floor or collapse on you it is so bad?

There are times I felt that worried about something to the point it made me feel that nervous and worked up and scared about it. All this is extremely traumatizing to me and it is very important to me that you tell me nothing is wrong well in advance.

## To Nurse Means To Nurture: Part Two

If I still continue to act scared you'll react badly to something, like a series of messages I sent you, if you only read some of them and not all of them and the thing I feared the worst might offend you that I said is something I'm not sure you saw, I'm still going to worry until I know for sure that the very thing I was the most scared of offending you with has not been read yet, because even though you told me you were not offended by the messages, the doubt still remains and I think, "What if they haven't read this message yet? They might not feel that way if they haven't read that yet?"

In some instances where I was that worried about something like this there really was something to worry about in those instances, but there have been many other instances where I might worry about the very same thing and find out after all my endless worry that the person read everything and they were never offended about anything to begin with.

I go to their office feeling like I'm about to face impending doom with a horrible stern lecture, which has happened before, and when I go in there the doctor or nurse might say, "What's the matter? Are you okay? Is something wrong?" and I might say, "I was scared to death if you saw this, or read this, or I said this to you that I would be in trouble for sure and you would hate me forever for it?" and that person might actually surprise me, which has also happened before and say, "No. You didn't offend me. I read everything and I wasn't offended about a thing. In fact, I thought you sounded cute."

I never know what to expect so when this happens I fear the worst and depending on the interpreter of what I said, if they didn't like what I said, I'm in big trouble, but if they liked what I said and thought it was cute, like a sweet person normally would think, I think, "What a relief! I was scared to death I ruined everything! I thought you would hate me forever! You're okay? You still like me? I guess everything was okay after all. That had me scared to death."

Most people would say, "That's too bad. None of this bothers me." It bothers me but it doesn't bother most people.

You may not feel like something I come up with that is not on my list of needs is not applicable to what you need to do for me but as far as the hugs, and the head rubs, and the hand holds and affection measures, which are on my list of needs are concerned those are dire needs I cannot do without and never could do without. Some of the other things I come up with off the cuff that are just hang-ups I have may drive me crazy too, yes, but the hugs, head rubs, and hand holds needs have to be met. I've needed all that from infancy to the present.

Please make sure to meet these needs whatever you do. Please do not let my other strange quirks stop you from doing those things I need most because I can't have it any other way. Thank you. Please keep reading.

Instead of looking at this section as being only about meeting my list of needs as a nurse and team of nurses like the first section in the book, you could look at it this way. This section would be more of a section on "Assurance of Forgiveness" in times of failure on the part of the patient when they have offended you.

So, if I ever offend you, please forgive me, and please assure me you will show me forgiveness and always be the way you always were and continue to meet my list of needs I have talked about in both of these books. Thank you.

The first section of this book before the one about my autism was more about "Assurance of Forgiveness" also, and about the "progression" from having a "nurse" as a "mother surrogate" to having a whole team of nurses as a "pseudo family". There was actually a quote about this very thing along with other quotes working up to it I got out of a college textbook of nursing I found.

Here is another quote regarding the relationship with a patient and their nurse practitioner who advocates for him:

"The interdependent relationship of the nursing and medical professions requires collaboration around the need of the client. The evolving role of the nurse in the health delivery system requires joint practice as colleagues, deliberations in determining functional relationships and differentiating areas of practice between the two professions."
    Basic Nursing: A Psychophysiologic Approach, Sorensen, Luckman, W.B. Saunders Company, 1979, page 354

My family doctor nurse practitioner does this for me when I go to other doctors and nurses at other doctor's offices such as walk in clinics and specialists and hospitals and I really appreciate it. Thank you for doing this for me.

"The nurse, in all professional relationships, practices with compassion and respect for the inherent dignity, worth, and uniqueness of every individual, unrestricted by considerations of social or economic status, personal attribute, or the nature of health problems. The nurse's primary commitment is to the client, whether an individual, family, group, or community. The nurse promotes, advocates for, and strives to protect the health, safety, and rights of the client."
    Fundamentals of Nursing, 7th Edition, Potter and Perry, Mosby Elsevier, 2009, page 315

The nurse needs to tell people what to expect of me and what my needs are so their will be no false judgment about me and all my childlike needs will be met like the hugs, head rubs, and hand holds, etc.

"The nurse is responsible and accountable for individual nursing practice and determines the appropriate delegation of tasks consistent with the nurse's obligation to provide optimum client care. The nurse owes the same duties to self as to others, including the responsibility to preserve integrity and safety, to maintain competence, and to continue personal and professional growth."
>Fundamentals of Nursing, 7th Edition, Potter and Perry, Mosby Elsevier, 2009, page 315

"The nurse participates in establishing, maintaining, and improving health care environments and conditions of employment conductive to the provision of quality health care and consistent with the values of the profession through individual and collective action. The nurse participates in the advancement of the profession through contributions to practice, education, administration, and knowledge development.
>Fundamentals of Nursing, 7th Edition, Potter and Perry, Mosby Elsevier, 2009, page 315

"The nurse collaborates with other health professionals and the public in promoting community, national, and international efforts to meet health needs."
>Fundamentals of Nursing, 7th Edition, Potter and Perry, Mosby Elsevier, 2009, page 315

The profession of nursing, as represented by associations and their members, is responsible for articulating nursing values, for maintaining the integrity of the profession and its practice and for shaping social policy."
>Fundamentals of Nursing, 7th Edition, Potter and Perry, Mosby Elsevier, 2009, page 315

"Nursing is a work of "intimacy". Nursing practice requires you to be in contact with clients not only physically but also emotionally, psychologically, and spiritually."
>Fundamentals of Nursing, 7th Edition, Potter and Perry, Mosby Elsevier, 2009, page 315

"In most other intimate relationships, you choose to enter the relationship precisely because you anticipate that your values will be shared with the other person. But in the case of nursing, you agree to provide care to your clients solely on the basis of their need for your services. Inevitably, you will work with clients whose values differ from yours. You will work with colleagues whose values differ from yours. To negotiate differences of opinion and value, it is important to have clarity about your own values: what you value, why, and how you respect your own values even as you try to respect those of others whose values differ from yours. A value is a personal belief about the worth of a given idea, attitude, custom, or object that sets standards that influence behavior."

>Fundamentals of Nursing, 7th Edition, Potter and Perry, Mosby Elsevier, 2009, page 315

"Professional nurses play a specific role in the management of health care. All clients in the health care system interact with a nurse at some point in ways that are unique to nursing. Nurses generally interact with clients over longer intervals of time than other disciplines. Because nurses are often involved in intimate physical acts such as bathing, feeding, and special procedures, clients and families reveal information not always shared with physicians, health care providers, or others.

>Fundamentals of Nursing, 7th Edition, Potter and Perry, Mosby Elsevier, 2009, page 319

"Details about family life, information about coping styles personal preferences, and details about fears and insecurities are likely to come out during the course of nursing interventions (Shannon, 1997)."

>Fundamentals of Nursing, 7th Edition, Potter and Perry, Mosby Elsevier, 2009, page 319

Remember, when you have to take care of me in this way, don't think of me as some stranger over here you're having to do this for and act defensive about having to do something like this for me because you think your professional somebody over here so I'd better not do anything wrong because you really didn't want to do this.

Think of me as a baby in diapers when you have to take care of me in this manner if this comes up and see me like I'm a little child you're giving a bath to if you have to give me a bath and try to be sweet about it. Other nurses have when they had to bathe me. I'm not just some intruder over here that you have to reluctantly give a bath that you have to be defensive with and act like I'm an adult and you're an adult so you'd better not do anything crazy. No, I'm a patient. Remember the quote in the first part of the book that said not to think of your patient as an intruder but as a person in need who needs your help and remember the other quote that says you need to let your patient's regress from their normal state and be allowed to act in childlike ways and be treated as a child.

That's what you are there for, not to condemn someone for having to give them a bath, but to offer your service to them when they do need a bath and talk sweetly to them like a mother talks to her little child. I don't understand why some people act this way.

Luckily the last couple of times I had to be given a bath or shaved for a procedure those girl nurses just saw me as a little kid who needed their service and did what they did for me with sweetness without complaining about anything because they felt like they wished they didn't have to do something like this. You're probably wondering, "Where did you get an idea like this from?"

Remember those ladies that complained about it 12 years ago and said I could do this my self if I wanted to? They complained about having to do it and acted all judgmental and then 3 days later they refused to let me take my own bath and insisted they were going to do it for me and they did. The whole thing was ridiculous.

They could have went in there and been nice about it and said, "Were you needing a bath today?" and I say, "Yes" and them say, "Okay here's what we need you to do in order to do this. Thankfully, the last two times since that I got a chipper acting, cheery female nurse to do it and they were very sweet about it and treated me like I was their little baby boy. That's the way it should be.

"Your ability to recognize these aspects of a client's situation and to express your professional concerns accordingly, will provide critical value to the discussion. The nursing point of view is part of a larger picture that includes all members of the health care team, including other providers of services and even the client and family."
>Fundamentals of Nursing, 7th Edition, Potter and Perry, Mosby Elsevier, 2009, page 319

"Many people with autism have sensory sensitivities, so that even basic health needs become an issue."
>Health Care and the Autism Spectrum, A Guide For Health Professionals, Parents and Carers, Alison Morton Cooper, Jessica Kingly Publishers, 2004, page24

"Pressures and stresses of 'trying to be normal' re-emerge, placing the child, young person or adult under yet more strain, with the risk of regression into withdrawal and the development of depression and anxiety disorders. The risk of suicide also increases, particularly where severe emotional problems are not recognized in time."
>Health Care and the Autism Spectrum, A Guide For Health Professionals, Parents and Carers, Alison Morton Cooper, Jessica Kingly Publishers, 2004, page27

I've felt pressured to be normal ever since I was taken out of special ed. I got treated horrible for my social differences. I couldn't hold down a job due to cluelessness in tasking and physical limitations.

I only did well in school in later years because of being drilled for hours on end for days on end just to pass my classes with Cs until I finally caught up with everybody else and starting making some As and Bs around a decade later only to find out I was too dumb to figure out how to perform various tasks at any of my jobs including manual labor jobs. This was especially my manual labor jobs as a matter of fact.

And then due to normalization I ask for certain special needs to be met as an adult by my nurses to meet my dire need for consistent hugs, and need for head rubs and hand holds through needle sticks because I seem normal to them and they think it is not in their job description to comfort their patients, especially by hugging them and touching them in any manner, which I proved them wrong about in my first "To Nurse Means to Nurture" book by the way, and I feel like a fish out of water because my interests are not the same as other guys and are more typical of little kids and girls than anything else.

Because I have difficulty getting my needs met I become depressed and when people refuse to meet my need for hugs, or the head rubs and hand holds through needle sticks to comfort me in my fear and pain, I actually lose my will to live and wish the end would get here.

"Professionals and the public need to understand that autism is life long even where it outwardly appears to be "mild". Support services and understanding need to be built around this."
> Health Care and the Autism Spectrum, A Guide For Health Professionals, Parents and Carers, Alison Morton Cooper, Jessica Kingly Publishers, 2004, page27

"Helping relationships are the foundation of clinical nursing practice. In such relationships, the nurse assumes the role of professional helper and comes to know the client as an individual who has "unique health needs", human responses, and patterns of living."
> Fundamentals of Nursing, 7th Edition, Potter and Perry, Mosby Elsevier, 2009, page 346

"The relationship is "therapeutic", promoting a psychological climate that facilitates positive change and growth. "Therapeutic communication" between the nurse and client allows the attainment of health-related goals (Arnold and Boggs, 2003). The goals of a "therapeutic relationship" focus on the client's achieving optimal personal growth (Stuart and Laraia, 2005)."
>Fundamentals of Nursing, 7th Edition, Potter and Perry, Mosby Elsevier, 2009, page 346

"There is and explicit time frame, a goal-directed approach, and a high expectation of confidentiality. The nurse establishes, directs, and takes responsibility for the interaction and the "clients needs take priority over the nurse's needs."
>Fundamentals of Nursing, 7th Edition, Potter and Perry, Mosby Elsevier, 2009, page 346

"The nurse's nonjudgmental acceptance of the client is an important characteristic of the relationship. Acceptance conveys a willingness to hear a message or to acknowledge feelings. It does not mean you always agree with the other person or approve of the client's decisions or actions. A helping relationship between nurse and client does not just happen – you create it with care, skill, and trust."
>Fundamentals of Nursing, 7th Edition, Potter and Perry, Mosby Elsevier, 2009, page 346

I need this acceptance no matter what I say or do that seem strange and I need to continue to receive the same comfort and the same friendly loving care I always received from my nurse when this does happen.

"Recently hospitalized clients described "emotional comfort" as a pleasant positive feeling and state of relaxation that resulted from "therapeutic interactions." Clients described emotional discomfort as unpleasant negative feelings and tension. Personal control over the situation contributed to emotional comfort. Clients perceived a positive link between emotional comfort and recovery."
>Fundamentals of Nursing, 7th Edition, Potter and Perry, Mosby Elsevier, 2009, page 347, Box 24-5

> I need as much love and affection and hugs you can give me because I am in dire need of all of this due to my Autism.

"Touch is a primal need, as necessary as food, growth or shelter. Think of "touch" as a nutrient transmitted through the skin and "skin hunger" as a form of malnutrition that has reached epidemic proportions in the United States, especially among older persons. Older adults need touch as much or more than any other age group. Simple touch helps older adult clients feel more connected to and accepted by those around them and to their environment."
> Fundamentals of Nursing, 7th Edition, Potter and Perry, Mosby Elsevier, 2009, page 784

I require a lot of attention and affection and I need you to touch me and I need you to give me hugs as well. As a nurse you are my "mother surrogate" while I am under your care and I expect these things to be done for me including every item on my lists of needs I have in both of these books. I expect all my nurses to be my "mother surrogates" that work with me and give me hugs and rub my head to calm me down and hold my hand through needle sticks to comfort me through the sticks as well as any other invasive procedures and wish to be put completely to sleep for any invasive procedures done on me. Because of my oversensitivity to pain remember to let me apply Lidocaine/Prilocaine 2.5% cream unless I don't have it on me, then apply it yourself 1 hour before a needle stick. I need chipper acting, cheery female nurses only. No serious trended female nurses and no male nurses or male techs.

Make sure to check on me often when I am an inpatient in the hospital and be sure to give me hugs every time and make sure I don't need you to comfort me in some way if I am anxious before any upcoming procedures.

## To Nurse Means To Nurture: Part Two

Try to cheer me up if I am sad or upset and keep me calm when I am scared and try to be there for me whenever I need you so I can feel less anxious and not feel lonely or abandoned if I have to wait long periods between things being done to me or if I am stuck in an inpatient ward for days on end or even one day and try to let me know if you're going to be going to a different floor if you are reassigned to a different ward because I will be continually nervous about you not coming back if you do because I will feel like I somehow did something wrong even when nothing is wrong and worry myself sick over it until you return.

If you can, do see if there is anyway they can let you be my nurse for the rest of the shift if you are someone I am really comfortable with so I don't feel dejected when they send someone else in there I may not really care for. It's happened before and I will think something is wrong if you don't tell me before you have to leave.

And, those of you assigning these nurses, please try to give me the most chipper acting ones you can find to give me and please try to fix it where they don't have to go to another floor in the middle of their shift. It would work better for me if the same nurse was able to stick around to wait on me for their entire shift than it would be to have them for two hours and then sorry, here comes Mrs. Blah to take their place. If they do have to leave, don't give me a blah acting female nurse replacement either. I need a chipper acting, cheery female nurse and they need to be as close to the same personality as the girl that left that I was comfortable with as possible. And, all my nurses need to give me hugs and rub my head to calm me down and hold my hand through any shots, blood tests, IVs, tube insertions, or anything else sharp or invasive that is painful to handle and scary to deal with.

Don't ever give me any male nurses or serious trended female nurses. I was tortured by those two kinds of nurses when I was a kid and if I ever get those kinds of nurses again you may not see me back again even if I have an emergency.

I will only cooperate with chipper acting; cheery female nurses and let them take care of me.

That is what I want and that is what I need. Thank you.

Also try to make sure I can get alternative foods for my meals because I am very picky and get grossed out very easily by various foods that don't taste right to me.

"Patients express frustration with the impersonal and diffuse care received in many large institutional settings. The nurse's focus should be on ensuring the preservation of personalism and continuity of care."
> Comprehensive Rehabilitation Nursing, Nancy Martin, Nancy B. Holt, Dorothy Hicks, McGraw Hill Book Company, 1981, page 569

"Hope and encouragement from the nurse can do much to raise the spirits of the patient and bolster efforts to continue living a fruitful life within the limitation of illness."
> Comprehensive Rehabilitation Nursing, Nancy Martin, Nancy B. Holt, Dorothy Hicks, McGraw Hill Book Company, 1981, page 569

"Providing presence is a person-to-person encounter conveying a closeness and a sense of caring.. Fredriksson (1999) explains that presence involves "being there" and "being with." "Being there is not only a physical presence, but also includes communication and understanding. The interpersonal relationship of "Being there" seems to depend on the fact that a nurse is attentive to the client (Cohen and others, 1994.) This type of presence is something the nurse offers to the client with the purpose of achieving some goal, such as support, comfort, or encouragement, to diminish the intensity of unwanted feelings, or for reassurance (Fareed, 1996; Pederson, 1993). Being with is also interpersonal."
> Fundamentals of Nursing, 7th Edition, Potter and Perry, page 100 & 101, Mosby Elsevier, 2009

"The nurse gives himself or herself, which means being available at and at a client's disposal (Pederson, 1993). If clients accept the nurse, they will invite him or her to see, share, and "touch" their vulnerability and suffering."
    Fundamentals of Nursing, 7th Edition, Potter and Perry,
    page 100 & 101, Mosby Elsevier, 2009

"One's human presence never leaves one unaffected (Watson, 2003). The nurse then enters the client's world. In this presence, the client is able to put words to feelings and to understand him self or her self in a way that leads to identifying solutions, seeing new directions, and making choices (Gilje, 1997). Establishing presence with a client enhances the nurse's ability to learn from the client. This strengthens the nurse's ability to provide adequate and appropriate nursing care."
    Fundamentals of Nursing, 7th Edition, Potter and Perry,
    page 100 & 101, Mosby Elsevier, 2009

"It is especially important to establish presence when clients are experiencing stressful events or situations."
    Fundamentals of Nursing, 7th Edition, Potter and Perry,
    page 100 & 101, Mosby Elsevier, 2009

"Awaiting a physician's report of test results, preparing for an unfamiliar procedure, and planning for a return home after serious illness are just a few examples of events in the course of a person's illness that can create unpredictability and dependency on care providers. The nurse's presence helps to calm anxiety and fear related to stressful situations."
    Fundamentals of Nursing, 7th Edition, Potter and Perry,
    page 100 & 101, Mosby Elsevier, 2009

"Giving reassurance and thorough explanations about a procedure, remaining at the client's side, and coaching the client through the experience all convey a presence that is invaluable to the client's well being."
    Fundamentals of Nursing, 7th Edition, Potter and Perry,
    page 100 & 101, Mosby Elsevier, 2009

"Clients face situations that are embarrassing, frightening, and painful. Whatever the feeling or symptom, clients look to nurse to proved comfort. The use of touch is one comforting approach where the nurse reaches out to clients to communicate concern and support. Touch is relational and leads to a connection between nurse and client. The skillful and gentle performance of a nursing procedure conveys security and a sense of competence. Caring touch is a form of nonverbal communication, which successfully influences a client's comfort and security, enhances self-esteem, and improves reality orientation (Boyek and Watson, 1994). You express this in the way you hold a client's hand, give a back massage, gently position a client, or participate in a conversation.
    Fundamentals of Nursing, 7th Edition, Potter and Perry, page 101, Mosby Elsevier, 2009

"When using a caring touch, the nurse is making a connection with the client and showing acceptance of the individual."
    Fundamentals of Nursing, 7th Edition, Potter and Perry, page 101, Mosby Elsevier, 2009

"Caring involves an interpersonal interaction that is much more than two persons simply talking back and forth. In a caring relationship the nurse establishes trust, opens lines of communication, and listens to what the client has to say (Figure 8-1). Listening is key, because it conveys the nurse's full attention and interest. Listening includes "taking in" what a client says, as well as an interpretation and understanding to the person talking (Kemper, 1992). Listening to the meaning of what a client says helps create a mutual relationship. True listening leads to truly knowing and responding to what really matters to the client and family (Boykin and others, 2003).
    Fundamentals of Nursing, 7th Edition, Potter and Perry, page 101, Mosby Elsevier, 2009

"When an ill person chooses to tell his or her story, it involves reaching out to another human being. Telling the story implies a relationship that develops only if the clinician exchanges his or her stories as well."
>	Fundamentals of Nursing, 7th Edition, Potter and Perry, page 102, Mosby Elsevier, 2009

"Through active listening, you begin to truly know your clients and what is important to them (Bernick, 2004).
>	Fundamentals of Nursing, 7th Edition, Potter and Perry, page 102, Mosby Elsevier, 2009

"The time you take to listen effectively is worthwhile both in the information gained and in the strengthening of the nurse-client relationships. Listening involves paying attention to the individual's words and tone of voice and entering his or her frame of reference."
>	Fundamentals of Nursing, 7th Edition, Potter and Perry, page 102, Mosby Elsevier, 2009

"By observing the expressions and body language of the client, you will find cues to help assist the client in exploring ways to achieve greater peace."
>	Fundamentals of Nursing, 7th Edition, Potter and Perry, page 102, Mosby Elsevier, 2009

"Knowing develops over time as a nurse learns the clinical conditions within a specialty and the behaviors and physiological responses of clients. Intimate knowing helps the nurse respond to what really matters to the client (Bulfin, 2005). To know a client means that the nurse "avoids assumptions", "focuses on the client", and "engages in a caring relationship" with the client that reveals information and cues that facilitate critical thinking and clinical judgments."
>	Fundamentals of Nursing, 7th Edition, Potter and Perry, page 102, Mosby Elsevier, 2009

## To Nurse Means To Nurture: Part Two

I really like it when my doctors and nurses listen to me and allow them to tell them anything that may be on my mind from a physical or emotional standpoint without judging me and seeing things for the way they are and not the way they might seem to be to them. When people consider my Autism things go way better. I'm sorry if I am offending anybody if you are someone who has never judged me before.

I have been in trouble so many times before mainly by people who never understood me in the first place, but I have been burned so many times before, even by people I thought understood me that I have this horrible fear that even if I don't consider you to be a judgmental person that if I say something that sounds too personal to you and you don't realize that it's just a little innocent "kid in a candy store" statement you might be shocked I said something you weren't expecting me to say and be forever upset thinking I meant something by it I never meant. Like I said, sometimes there are things that bug me I feel like I've just got to have a certain way or I've just got to ask because I feel like I'm just going to bust if I can't get it that are coming from the emotional standpoint of a kindergartner but they may sound some other way because normal people might have a different reason for wanting the same thing.

"Knowing the client is at the core of the process nurses use to make clinical decisions. By establishing a caring relationship, the understanding that develops helps the nurse to better know the client as a unique individual and choose the most appropriate efficacious nursing therapies."
   Fundamentals of Nursing, 7th Edition, Potter and Perry, page 102, Mosby Elsevier, 2009

"The caring relationships that a nurse develops over time, compiled with the nurse's growing knowledge and experience, provide a rich source of meaning when changes in a client's clinical status occur."
   Fundamentals of Nursing, 7th Edition, Potter and Perry, page 102, Mosby Elsevier, 2009

"The experienced nurse knows additional facts about his or her clients such as their experiences, behaviors, feelings, and perceptions (Radwin, 1995)."
>   Fundamentals of Nursing, 7th Edition, Potter and Perry, page 102, Mosby Elsevier, 2009

"When you make clinical decisions accurately in the context of knowing a client well, improved client outcomes will result. Swanson (1999b) notes that when nurses base care on knowing the client, the clients perceive care as "personalized", "comforting", "supporting", and "healing".
>   Fundamentals of Nursing, 7th Edition, Potter and Perry, page 102, Mosby Elsevier, 2009

"Success in knowing the client lies in the relationship you establish. To know a client is to enter into a caring, social process that result in a "bonding" whereby the client comes to feel known by the nurse (Lamb and Stempel, 1994" The "bonding" then sets the stage for the relationship to evolve into working and changing phases so that you help the client become involved in his or her care and accept help when needed (Bulfin, 2005)."
>   Fundamentals of Nursing, 7th Edition, Potter and Perry, page 101, Mosby Elsevier, 2009

"If health care is to make positive differences in their lives, human beings cannot be treated like "machines" or "robots". Instead, "Health care" has to become more "humanizing". Nurses play an important role in making "care" an integral part of health care delivery. This begins by nurses making "caring" a part of the philosophy and environment in the workplace. Incorporating care concepts into standards of nursing care establishes the guidelines for professional conduct. Finally, during the day-to-day practice with clients and families, nurses need to be committed to caring and be willing to establish the relationships necessary for personal competent, compassionate and meaningful care."
>   Fundamentals of Nursing, 7th Edition, Potter and Perry, page 103, Mosby Elsevier, 2009

"For the person affected by autism, even a typically doctor consultation or visit to the practice nurse can be traumatic and anxiety – provoking experience with unlimited outcomes for those involved"
> Health Care and the Autism Spectrum, A Guide For Health Professionals, Parents and Carers, Alison Morton Cooper, Jessica Kingly Publishers, 2004, page23

My newest family doctor, nurse practitioner has done very well with me and I hope that never changes. I love my newest family doctor, nurse practitioner and I hope she still loves me. Many others have been difficult to work with and did not understand my needs. It would be horrible if I said or did anything to turn my favorite nurse practitioner away because she has been very sweet to me and meets my needs very well and advocates for me to others to help them understand me so they will do the same. I don't ever want to ruin that. She is very special to me and she is like a "mother" figure to me. She is the sweetest, most wonderful doctor I have ever had or met. I hope she always stays that way.

"Communicating with a person who has autism can be a profound learning experience for those who take the time to value its lessons and can teach a great deal about the intricacies of the practitioner-patient relationship."
> Health Care and the Autism Spectrum, A Guide For Health Professionals, Parents and Carers, Alison Morton-Cooper, Jessica Kingsley Publishers, 2004, page 36

"This risks involved are very real. First there is the risk that the patient may be misunderstood or have their needs misinterpreted. Then there is the risk of misdiagnosis resulting from poor-quality communication."
> Health Care and the Autism Spectrum, A Guide For Health Professionals, Parents and Carers, Alison Morton Cooper, Jessica Kingly Publishers, 2004, page23

Sometimes I say things or ask things out of innocence that may sound odd in nature and can be interpreted as being something totally the opposite of what it sounds like.

## To Nurse Means To Nurture: Part Two

I may want what I am asking for, but the motive for asking whatever it is I am asking for is purely out of innocence and not mischievousness. If a normal person were to ask the same thing for mischievous reasons I fear if I ask for the same thing out of innocence that I may be scolded for asking for things of a mischievous nature, not thinking the mischievous thoughts they may think I am thinking and be in serious trouble for something that isn't even what it looks like and be lucky I don't lose a friend. I hope if this ever happens I receive forgiveness and reassurance and I also hope something happens to reveal to this person that what I wanted was out of innocence and not mischievousness. I waited way too long to have this good a thing and I don't want to ruin it. If only I could be free to say whatever stupid things I think of to say or ask without having to worry about being judged for what a normal person thinks when they make the same requests things would be a lot better anywhere. I'm an ex-special ed student. Please. Before you condemn me for something that isn't even the case, think to yourself, "What would a special ed person mean if they asked me this? What would they mean if they said this? What would a little kid mean if they asked me this? What would they mean if they said this? Why would a little kid want he is asking me for? What would a Special Ed person want he is asking me for? Is my patient with autism that tends to act like a 5 year old already even if he is an adult just acting like a kindergartner again? Is he thinking what they are thinking? Is he having their kind of emotions when he asks me this? Why would a kindergartner ask me if I would do this for them? Why would a kindergartner say something strange like this to me?
You know that kids can come up with some of the most off the wall questions you ever heard of and say some of the most shocking things you ever heard, but you know they don't mean anything by it and they are just thinking like a bunch of kindergartners don't you? If only I could get you to believe me, a lot of the things I say or ask for that sound odd or even outlandish to some people is nothing more than a statement based on the emotion a kindergartner would have that would set them off to ask you the strange question they ask you where they either ask you to do the oddest things for them or make the oddest statements or requests. You know they don't mean any harm by it don't you?

Neither do I.

I may be intellectually an adult, but socially and emotionally I am just like them and people have even told Bertha they felt like dealing with me was like taking care of a kindergartner before because I get mixed up over the strangest things and say some of the oddest stuff and ask the strangest questions you ever heard and it all sounds to them like the equivalent of that of what a kindergartner would say, do, or ask.

But, when people do not see this fact, I say something the least bit odd, and slam I'm in serious trouble for something I said because they think I meant something that I never meant and they jump down my throat and give me a stern lecture and try to scold me for inappropriate behaviors, not because they were inappropriate but because they interpreted them as being inappropriate based on what normal people mean when they say or ask the same things.

Please, when you base judgment on what I say when I say odd things, don't hold me up to the standards of the normal world, and don't assume I meant what an individual from the normal world meant if they would ask the same thing of you for all the wrong reasons.

Instead, base your judgment on what a Special Ed person would think and feel when they ask you strange things or what a little kid or even a kindergartner would ask you for that matter, because like them, believe it or not I have a lot of the same feelings they do with their emotions and their desires and I tend to want and need things from people that would normally be considered strange from someone else and be regarded as something bad but yet would be totally innocent from the heart of a child or a kindergartner or a Special Ed student, so when you base judgment on what I say when something sounds odd, don't base it on what the normal world means but base it on what a kindergartner would mean and what the Special Ed world would mean.  Thank you.

"Autism in all its forms is a complex, lifelong neurodevelopmental disorder that can profoundly affect a person's ability to communicate with, and understand the behaviors of those around them. People with autism find it difficult to communicate their thoughts, feelings, and physical sensations in ways that are easy for others to understand; this can render them very vulnerable when illness strikes, or when normal physical development demands attention."

> Health Care and the Autism Spectrum, A Guide For Health Professionals, Parents and Carers, Alison Morton Cooper, Jessica Kingly Publishers, 2004, page22

This is a big problem with me and this is why I've written so much to my doctors in the past trying to explain what my medical problems are and what they entail with the multiple symptoms that arise with them.

I also feel like I have to over explain myself when expressing my feelings about things in fear someone might mistake something for something bad a normal person would have meant when my reasoning for the same thing is of an innocent nature or I am affected totally different from the everyday person by the same things.

I fear I will be judged for thinking things I do not think based on things I say or ask for and receive a stern lecture for it and get the cold shoulder treatment where I will be lucky if that particular doctor ever treats me the same again due to misunderstandings where if they would have seen it in the eyes of someone observing a child asking the same things they would see the difference and realize there was never any harm meant at all. If something ever sounds strange to you that I come up with it's probably not what it sounds like.

I can say things sometimes that can be easily misinterpreted as being mischievous in nature if you are looking at it from the perspective of what a normal person would mean by what I said, but if you took the same statement from the standpoint of a disabled person with the mind of a child saying the same thing or asking the same thing from the standpoint of a 5 year old then you can suddenly see just how innocent it is what they just said when you take what they said from their own perspective rather than that of a normal person's perspective. So please keep that in mind when I say anything odd or ask anything odd of you. I'm probably thinking from the perspective of a child when I do this and it might as well have been a 5 year old that said or asked you the same thing because I have the socialization of a 5 year old. So please accept me the way I am and continue to be my nurse.

"Caring is the heart of a nurse's ability to work with people in a respectful and therapeutic way."
>Fundamentals of Nursing, 7th Edition, Potter and Perry, page 103, Mosby Elsevier, 2009

"Caring is specific and "relational" for each "nurse-client relationship".
>Fundamentals of Nursing, 7th Edition, Potter and Perry, page 103, Mosby Elsevier, 2009

My newest family doctor, female nurse practitioner is really good with this and is better with me than anyone I've ever had.

"For caring to achieve cure, nurses need to learn those culturally specific behaviors and words that reflect human caring in different cultures."
>Fundamentals of Nursing, 7th Edition, Potter and Perry, page 103, Mosby Elsevier, 2009

"Because illness is the human experience of loss or dysfunction, any treatment or intervention given without consideration of its meaning to the individual is likely to be worthless."
>Fundamentals of Nursing, 7th Edition, Potter and Perry, page 103, Mosby Elsevier, 2009

"Swanson's theory of caring includes five caring processes: "knowing", "being with", "doing for", "enabling", and "maintaining belief".
>Fundamentals of Nursing, 7th Edition, Potter and Perry, page 104, Mosby Elsevier, 2009

"Caring involves a mutual give and take that develops as nurse and client begin to "know and care for one another".
>Fundamentals of Nursing, 7th Edition, Potter and Perry, page 104, Mosby Elsevier, 2009

"It is difficult to show caring to individuals without gaining an understanding of "who they are" and "their perception of their illness".
>Fundamentals of Nursing, 7th Edition, Potter and Perry, page 104, Mosby Elsevier, 2009

"Presence involves a person-to-person encounter that conveys a "closeness" and a "sense of caring" that involves "being there" and "being with" clients".
>Fundamentals of Nursing, 7th Edition, Potter and Perry, page 104, Mosby Elsevier, 2009

"Research shows that "touch", both contact and noncontact, includes "task orientated touch", "caring touch", and "protective touch."
>Fundamentals of Nursing, 7th Edition, Potter and Perry, page 104, Mosby Elsevier, 2009

"The skillful and "gentle performance" of a nursing procedure conveys security and a sense of competence in the nurse."
>Fundamentals of Nursing, 7th Edition, Potter and Perry, page 104, Mosby Elsevier, 2009

"Listening is not only "taking in " what a client says, it also includes interpretation and understanding of what the cline is saying and giving back that understanding to the person talking."
>Fundamentals of Nursing, 7th Edition, Potter and Perry, page 104, Mosby Elsevier, 2009

"Knowing the client is at the core of the process nurses use to make clinical decisions."
>Fundamentals of Nursing, 7th Edition, Potter and Perry, page 104, Mosby Elsevier, 2009

"Nurses demonstrate "caring" by helping family members become more active participants in a client's care."
>Fundamentals of Nursing, 7th Edition, Potter and Perry, page 104, Mosby Elsevier, 2009

"Nursing the patient with autism well, therefore draws on this kind of engagement with practice and with the moral endeavor to do what is best in the interest of the patient given their needs and personal aspirations."
>Health Care and the Autism Spectrum, A Guide For Health Professionals, Parents and Carers, Alison Morton-Cooper, page 85, Jessica Kingsley Publishers, 2004

"Patients will normally need to be cared for by at least two nursing staff together if they are febrile and unwell, for they may be very restless and agitated and unable to understand what is being done to help them."
>Health Care and the Autism Spectrum, A Guide For Health Professionals, Parents and Carers, Alison Morton-Cooper, page 94, Jessica Kingsley Publishers, 2004

"If catherization is required because of urinary problems or surgery, special care will be needed to see that this is carried out as gently as possible or it is likely to cause extreme distress. Similarly, any invasive procedure, such as inserting chest or wound drains or cleaning wounds and attending to pressure area care, will require very sensitive and minimal handling and close observation."
>Health Care and the Autism Spectrum, A Guide For Health Professionals, Parents and Carers, Alison Morton-Cooper, page 94, Jessica Kingsley Publishers, 2004

"Autism is a lifelong condition characterized by an abnormality of brain function leading to difficulties in communicating with and understanding the intentions of others."

> Health Care and the Autism Spectrum, A Guide For Health Professionals, Parents and Carers, Alison Morton-Cooper, page 26, Jessica Kingsley Publishers, 2004

"Carers and families need support not only during a period of hospitalization for their relative with autism, but also day to day living. Staff working in community or residential settings recognize that working with people with autism can be draining physically and emotionally but also very rewarding. They also know, however, that (residential core workers excepted) they can go home at the end of their shift or working hours and recoup energy given up at work."

> Health Care and the Autism Spectrum, A Guide For Health Professionals, Parents and Carers, Alison Morton-Cooper, page 94, Jessica Kingsley Publishers, 2004

Now let's take all this and put it into action. Let's assume a patient has a 3 day stay in the hospital as an inpatient or even longer. Let's see how we can personalize the care we give them in each thing that we do as we nurse them throughout the day every day.

For me, as I said, I need chipper acting female nurses only to give me hugs and rub my head to calm me down through needle sticks.

Make sure I never get a male nurse or a serious trended female nurse. See to it that the chipper acting female nurses I do get check on me regularly, preferably once every 20 to 30 minutes.

I need hugs from these nurses every time I see them when they come in and when they leave. Remember, I found a quote that says you guys are supposed to allow me to regress and be allowed to act in childlike ways and ask you to meet childlike requests, which are also dire needs of mine. I require a lot of attention and a lot of affection. I am a very clingy person and always require lots of hugs.

I already have a regressed frame of mind anyway due to Autism.

If I appear sad or upset or scared it would be nice if you went in and rubbed my shoulder or my head and said, "Are you okay? Here, let me stay with you a minute and help you calm down." like you would a little child or a little boy. You might hold my hand every now and then, but always give me hugs when you come in and when you leave.

And, if I'm really upset and feel like I have to cry or something you might hold me a minute and hug me until I have a chance to cry it out if I am upset about something.

If you come in to adjust the room temperature for example, instead of just manually adjusting the air and not saying another word, be personal about it. When you adjust the air, come in and sweetly ask, "I was going to come in to adjust the temperature of your room. Do you feel warm? Do you need me to turn the air on? I thought you might like some cool fresh air. Would you like me to turn the cooler on? Are you cold? Do you need me to turn the temperature up? Would you like me to turn it up or down?" You might come in ever so often and say, "Would you like something to drink?" in a sweet tone of voice. And nicely take whatever cups I have and fill them up with water and coffee and come back in yourself and not someone else unless you just flat can't get to me.

But, please try to come back in yourself if you are the main one taking care of me because it makes me nervous when you ask me something like that and run off and send someone else in the room. I get worried really easily when this happens and think I must have said or done something wrong to offend you. If I ever do offend you, it's usually completely unintentional. They only way it would be intentional is if you said something to make me mad because I thought you were being harsh with me and I was upset about it. Otherwise, if it's just some trivial thing, even if it sounds personal then no offense is ever meant because I like nice people and I like to be as nice to them as I possibly can and be sweet back to sweet acting people because that's just my personality.

## To Nurse Means To Nurture: Part Two

It doesn't mean anything bad when I do that.

That's just me, because whatever I said is probably coming from the mind of a child where I meant the same thing some little kid would have said if I said it rather than some normal adult over here. If you ever are offended by anything I say or do then please forgive me and continue to treat me like you always have because it's probably not what it looks like when you take something wrong I say or do or I probably don't even realize what I said.
If something ever does happen I should actually need assistance with toileting, please just sweetly guide me into the bathroom and help me on to the toilet and help me with sitting and standing and holding the toilet paper if needed and do what you need to do and nicely stand me up as gently and easily as you possibly can trying to do your best not to jerk the tubes around such as IVs or catheters when you walk me in there, help me down, help me up and help me back to my bed. If I need help with dressing then help me pull my pants up and guide me to my bed if you need to. But guide me gently and act friendly to me and talk sweetly to me when you do and when you help me into the bed give me a hug when you put me back to bed and make sure I don't need anything else while your still there like drinks or food or snacks. Thank you.
I'm not meaning to sound inappropriate here or gross you out or embarrass you. I just want to be treated personally and not like a machine you want to move around as quickly as you can and dump off somewhere because you don't want to be personal with me.
As odd as this may sound, just like the other stuff I am asking you to do personally, this is called "palliative care". There are certain hospitals that already use this type of care, but typically this type of care should be shown to patients at every hospital. Sorry if I just embarrassed you. It's a little odd talking about toileting, and I doubt seriously you ever have to do this for me anytime soon unless I'm having a really horrible time getting around by myself in a hospital and am that bad off. Most people have not had to do this for me. Nurses have had to assist me to the bathroom before and told me to call them when I was done. I had some difficult even walking to the sink to wash my hands. I always tried to make it anyway and washed my hands and then I'd call them to help me.

I don't think you're really supposed to do that but I wanted to save them the extra trouble. When I called them, they came for me and helped me back to my bed.

If it's time for bedtime and you want to go in to turn off lights and you want to know whether to turn them off or not or which ones, come in and sweetly ask "Would you like me to turn these lights out? I'm getting everybody ready for bed because it's time to go to sleep. Would you like me to turn the night light on or the desk lamp on for you or would you like them turned off? Is there anything I can get you? Do you need anything else to drink? Do you need any more blankets or any more pillows I can get you?" And if there is any more blankets I need then please put the blanket over me and put the pillow under my head and adjust it and tuck me in and give me a hug and tell me goodnight.

I know this probably sounds silly or you might think, "This is ridiculous. I'm not your mother. I'm a nurse." But the nurses are supposed to take the place of your mother and I'm a clingy person and I always cling to my mother even now when I go see her.

So, I want to be treated like I'm your sweet little baby boy your tucking in for bed to say goodnight because I'm your patient and your like a mother to me.

I need hugs when you come in to check my vitals too and also when you bring me drinks. I don't mean to be a burden. I'm just a clingy person and I need a lot of affection and attention and I have a dire need for attention and affection and always have had a dire need to receive affection and attention my whole life because I am actually a special needs person and my autism causes me to be this way.

When someone comes in to adjust my IV, or if you're the one doing it either one, I need you to come in and say, "I'm coming in to adjust your IV. I'll be as gentle as possible so don't be scared okay." and then you could gently pat my hand or arm or shoulder and then give me a hug and say, "There. That wasn't so bad was it?"

When you come into give me a bath, I want you to treat me like a baby in diapers and still be sweet to me and be as motherly as you can when you do it as if you're giving a bath to your own little boy.

Don't think of me as some intruder that you have to scold for giving me a bath, just do it like you enjoy doing it for the sake of taking care of a special person with special needs who needs your help that might as well be a child themselves even if they are an adult.

Please don't ever be afraid to look at anything if I need to show you something. I'm not going to show you anything you don't want to see unless I really think that something is wrong. For example, if I have a rash and I need you to look at it and see if there is something you can do for it, once again, don't treat me like an intruder you have to scold for inappropriateness because I'm asking you to look at a rash. A rash is a rash and you're a nurse and sometimes nurses have to see things they really don't want to see.

I don't want to intentionally embarrass you but when things come up where a nurse has to do what a nurse has to do and it means they have to look at something private in order to do it that's just the way it goes because that's your job and that is what you are there for. If you're wondering why I'm even suggesting a nurse might be scolding for something like this in this manner it's because 20 years ago, I did have a rash, and in fear the nurses would think I was being inappropriate for bringing it to their attention I let it go for 2 months and it got worse and worse and worse. When I finally did get up the nerve to tell the nurses I was going to about the rash they got really upset and talked to each other in front of me like "Why did we have to get stuck looking at this?" complaining about it. They saw a rash alright and it was bad but they were upset about having to look at it because they had to see my private area in order to take care of it. They got the head nurse and said, "I think you need to look at this! This is bad!"

The head nurse said, "It's bad alright!" Put this type of cream over here on it that's in this big, long tube bottle and smear it on their good and see if that takes care of it and give him some more to take home with him. We'll have to get him a prescription."
You would be surprised what all I've gotten in trouble for even when something was really wrong that needed to be taken care of just because someone didn't want to have to look at something they didn't want see.

I know you're thinking, "Why don't you get a guy to do it?" but I don't care, I want a female nurse to do everything with me I don't care what they have to see. I don't care if they have to give me a bath or take care of a rash or anything like that. I want them to take care of it and them only.

I want the chipper acting female nurses for everything, including the baths and all the private care. I want you to be my mothers and work with me like I'm your own little boy you sweetly want to take care of and I want you to do everything that has to be done both private and non private.

Please give me hugs when you come in to take my vitals. There are usually two or three that come in together for that and I need all of you that come in to give me hugs and I need all of you to be "chipper acting, cheery female nurses" and not "serious trended" female nurses, no matter who you are or what you are doing. That goes for RNs, LPNs, Radiology Techs, Anesthesiologists, Lab Techs, CNAs, ER techs, Cardiology nurses, Respiratory Techs, all of you. No "male" nurses and no "serious trended" female nurses. Happy go lucky, chipper acting, cheery female nurses only allowed. Thank you.

Please give me hugs before and after you leave when you give me my medicine at pill time too.

When someone comes to put my IV in I need one of you to do the IV stick while the other one rubs my head to calm me down and holds my hand.

## To Nurse Means To Nurture: Part Two

When someone comes to remove my IV I need one of you to pull the IV out as gently as possible while the other one rubs my head to calm me down and holds my hand.

Both of you doing this have to be chipper acting, cheery female nurses only and both of you need to give me lots of hugs.

I'm very needy, and you are suppose to let me regress and let you take care of me like a child and you guys could be like mommies to me and when I'm scared it would be like, "Its okay. Mommy's here. Hold on to me. You're going to be okay. We're going to get you through this. Okay. You just wait and see."

If something happens any of you need to reinsert my IV, I need one chipper acting; cheery female nurse to reinsert the IV while another chipper acting, cheery female nurse rubs my head to calm me down and holds my hand again. Also give me lots of hugs before and after you are done and let me hold on to you when I am scared and let me cry on you if I need to. I am a very needy person. I am actually very vulnerable and gullible and some people can see that right away but others can't always see it right off the bat until they get around me a while.

When they figure it out after not believing me when they finally figure it out it's usually too late when they do figure it out because complete disaster happens and then they wish they would have intervened like they should have instead of assuming I was somebody just trying to play games with them about my needs. My needs have always been there and my needs are genuine. The only reason some of you cannot see them is because I was taken out of Special Ed and normalized for so many years that you usually can't tell it until you get around me a while and then the light comes on, "Something's not right. This guy's not all there. Someone might take advantage of him." Because I was normalized and this normalization has blinded everyone to my true needs it leaves me susceptible to evil people to take advantage of me because everyone else assumes my needs are a joke until they find out all too late that I was never joking in the first place.

I wish I would have never been taken out of Special Ed in the first place and then I wouldn't have this problem and everyone would see it from the start and act accordingly because they would know it wasn't a joke, that my needs are genuine and my needs are for real.

I'm sorry I ever left that world. I didn't ask to be taken out of there. I just was. And, now look at how misinterpreted I get because of it.

If anybody comes at me with blades or scalpels or tubes or biopsies I also need one chipper acting female nurse to use the instruments to do what they wish to accomplish while another chipper acting female nurse rubs my head to calm me down and holds my hand and I want lots of hugs from both of you.
For all invasive procedures I need to be sent to pre-op and put completely to sleep for you do perform them.

When you bring my meals please help me set them up on the table so I can get to everything easily. Also, please make sure to see if there are any alternative meals and bring me a menu to look at to see if there is something better I'd like than what you are serving.

Check regularly to see if I need coffee, water, or soda, because I drink a lot, especially water, but I drink a lot of coffee and soda too, and I snack a lot.

Always make sure to give me hugs when you come in and go out to do this.

When you help me brush my teeth, please help hold the plastic thing under me while I brush and put the toothpaste on my brush if I am unable to get out of bed while I brush my teeth. If I can get up and go to the sink I'll probably do it myself, but if I am having trouble standing for some reason you might try to hold me up when you do it.

Be sure to be gentle with me when getting me in and out of bed to go to the bathroom or eat or walk or anything else.

## To Nurse Means To Nurture: Part Two

Be gentle with the way you move the IV around and try not to pull on it too much. If I have a catheter in me and you get me in and out of bed please move me around in bed as gently as possible and move the catheter out of the way as gently as possible without yanking it.

And, if you are just going into the room to adjust the catheter, please be gentle with how you pull it and do it very gradually and easily. Try not to jerk or yank on the catheter. Others have done this to me before and put me in excruciating pain.

I also want to be able to go up to the nurses' station every now in then when I feel well enough to get up and around to give everybody else hugs too.

And, the rest of you nurses don't be so impersonal yourselves either because you are like my "pseudo family" of "surrogate mothers" while I am in the hospital and I need all of you to be my "surrogate mothers." Make sure to always hug me hello and hug me goodbye, all of you. And, I usually need a few more hugs from everybody in between because I'm a really clingy person who is needy that has special needs I need met because of my Autism.

Please make sure to always give me plenty of hugs, head rubs, and hand holds and shoulder pats, etc. I need all the affection I can get. If there ever comes a time when a relative dies that I am close to and I am grieved by it I need you to hug me and hold me while I cry on you and show me as much affection as you possibly can and do everything you can to cheer me up and make me feel better. My mother will probably only make it another 5 or 6 years at the most because people in my family only tend to live up to their early to mid 80s. My grandmother on her side was 84 when she died and my grandfather on her side was only 79 when he died. My mother just turned 79 this past December, so I need you to be ready to be there for me if anything ever happens to her.
And, to my sweet, family doctor, female nurse practitioner I need you to be there for me when this happens.

## To Nurse Means To Nurture: Part Two

I know you're not in Texas and she is, but if I go down there for a period at the time something should happen and come back up at the time something of this nature should occur, I need you to hold on to me and hug me and let me cry on you when she does go. Please. You're so sweet; I figured you would have no trouble with this. I've also asked the same thing of one of my favorite church members and they will be there for me too and let me cry on them too.

I need chipper acting female nurses and chipper acting female friends that I have to all be there for me to do this for me, but especially the ones that I am closest to. Please be willing to do this for me and please do not be upset that I asked. I really need this badly and I don't think I could make it without your help because it needs to be people I feel the closest to and look up the most to that do this for me, but even if I do barely know you and you are a nurse, if you are sweet and I like you I want to be able to do this with you too. Please and thank you.

                Your friend,
                Brian Gene Evans

# To Nurse Means To Nurture: Part Two

Dear Nurses,

Please note my needs when you take care of me. I appear to be normal but I am actually autistic and have childlike needs. I need a lot of affection from cheery acting, chipper female nurses with motherly personalities who are caring and compassionate and willing to comfort me the way I ask them to comfort me. I have a sensory issue in my right ear that can only be relieved by putting my right ear on the cheek of the people I like, I call doing this a hug. So, I need to be able to do this with my nurses as well to bring me comfort, especially in medical situations, and I need to do it even worse when I'm scared. A cheery acting female nurse also needs to rub the top of my head and hold my hand to comfort me through an IV stick, blood test or shot, while another cheery acting female nurse does the stick. They also need to do this for me if I have a biopsy awake or have to be stuck with or cut with any other sharp instruments. It is really important I have these met. Those who have done this for me in the past did really well with me. I have a fear of needles and oversensitivity to pain. A shot and a blood test feel like being stuck with a steak knife. An IV feels like being stabbed with a butcher knife. A catheter feels like a sword being run through me. I need to be able to put Lidocaine/Prilocaine 2.5% cream on the site of the stick because of this. I need to be knocked out for all invasive procedures, as well as any catheter or tube insertions. I also need all the radiology techs and anesthesiologists and everybody that deals with me needs to be cheery, chipper acting females only and I need to be able to put my right ear on their cheek too because of my sensory issue. Male doctors, nurses, and techs tortured me as a child so I am scared of men. The serious trended female nurses also tortured me in childhood and adulthood so I am scared of them too. Please give me chipper acting, cheery female nurses to work with me only.

To Nurse Means To Nurture: Part Two

Dear Nurses,

For those of you who are unable to catch what all of my needs are on the letter you just saw who need to see them in list form, here is my list of needs again. Please meet all these needs on this list. Not doing so traumatizes me, so it's very important you meet these.

- Need All Chipper Acting, Cheerful Female Nurses Only
- No Male Nurses, Therapists, Techs, Radiologists, or Anesthesiologists
- No Serious Trended Female Nurses, Therapists, Techs, Radiologists, or Anesthesiologists
- Need Hugs from All My Nurses (A Hug to Me is Putting my Right Ear on Your Cheek)
- Need a Chipper Acting, Cheerful Female Nurse to Rub my Head to Calm me Down and Hold my Hand While Another Chipper Acting Female Nurse does the IV, Blood Test, or Shot
- They Also Need To Do This For Me If Any Biopsies are taken awake, or any Blades, Or Scalpels, or Other Sharp Instruments Are Used On Me Awake
- I Need to Be Able to Put on Lidocaine/Prilocaine 2.5% Cream on Site of Stick
One Hour Before A Needle Stick of Any Kind
- Need to Be Knocked Out For Any Catheter Insertions or Tube Insertions
(Heart or Urinary Catheter Insertions)
* Need to Be Able to Write Doctors/Nurses About Any Medical Conditions/Symptoms   I Have or Any Emotional Needs I  Need Met
* Need All Medical Professionals Dealing With Me to Be Informed of the Needs
On this List and Be Willing to Meet Them

You meet this list and we are good to go. I still need to hug everyone I see so don't just limit it to one or two people that specifically work with me.

## To Nurse Means To Nurture: Part Two

I need to be able to hug everybody I see when I go for a test in the Radiology Department for example, or the Pre-Op Department for example. Being able to do this helps me to be able to feel safe in my environment and comfortable with my nurses with the reassurance that anyone who does any other test on me in the same department will always be the same way with me as well as the ones that work with me, but do still only give me the chipper acting female nurses only to work with me because they are the nurses I am comfortable with. Plus, I have a sensory issue in my right ear that can only be relieved by being able to place my right ear on the cheek of all the people I like, including nurses. Not only that, but there are some tests that are so difficult for me to handle you may need extra assistance at times as well, so it is also better that everybody be prepared to give me a hug so I can feel at ease with everyone and know I will be taken care of in the way I need cared for with the comfort I need to receive from them in the way I need to receive it from them and not by what they decide but by how I tell them they need to comfort me, by giving me hugs, let me press my right ear on their cheek, and rub my head to calm me down and hold my hand through needle sticks. I need chipper acting cheery female nurses only to work with me.

The chipper acting cheery female nurses are the most compassionate people that do better at comforting me and making me feel at ease than anyone else. Male nurses and serious trended nurses tortured me as a child. Serious trended female nurses also tortured me as an adult. I need the chipper acting female nurses only to work with me that have cheery motherly personalities and comfort me the way I state I need comforted and I will be good to go. I am autistic and have childlike needs and need to be comforted in the way I ask to be comforted because this is the only thing that works for me. Please see to it that this is done for me, and we're set to go. Thank you.

Your friend,

Brian Gene Evans

Also available are:

"Big City Hospitals Don't Like Cowards: A view of the Nursing World by an Autistic Man" by Brian Gene Evans

"To Nurse Means to Nurture: The Need For Nurses to Comfort their Patients" by Brian Gene Evans

"Mainstreaming a Disabled Person into the Normal World is a Big Mistake" by Brian Gene Evans

"What Language Therapy Really Entails" by Brian Gene Evans

"Compassion for Disabled Peers is Needed in College"
By Brian Gene Evans

"Autism Undiagnosed: What Happened?" by Bertha Marie Evans

"Autism Undiagnosed Part Two: Will I Always be an Outcast"
By Bertha Marie Evans

"Joys and Sorrows of Living with Adult Autism" by Bertha Marie Evans

"Victory" by Bertha Marie Evans

"How to Have a Happy Marriage" by Bertha Marie Evans


To contact us if you have any questions or would like Bertha to do a talk on Autism, Addictions, or Abuse at your facility you can call us at (870) 416–1030.

If no one is there, simply leave us a message on our phone and we will get back with you as soon as possible. Thank you.

Your friend,

Brian Gene Evans

www.ingramcontent.com/pod-product-compliance
Lightning Source LLC
Chambersburg PA
CBHW060418190526
45169CB00002B/963